Praise from Health Professi

"I highly recommend Dr. Lau's natural scoliosis program as .... effective alternative to the conventional bracing and surgery that is commonly recommended. I am very impressed with the results I have seen! I think that every spinal specialist needs this information."

— *Dr. Alan Kwan, D.O. Medical Director*

"As an Orthopaedic Surgeon, I usually recommend surgical treatments for scoliosis as the last recourse. Most scoliosis sufferers do not meet the parameters of a surgical candidate and should seek more conservative measures. Dr. Lau's program is a safe and painless alternative for scoliosis patients and has merit. I would recommend trying Dr. Lau's non-surgical scoliosis correction program."

— *Dr. Gul Keng, M.D. Orthopaedic Surgeon*

Testimonials From Patients

"Dr. Kevin Lau presents the facts in a logical and rational sequence. I appreciated that his tips were easy to follow and relatively fuss-free. It did not require me to spend extra time, efforts and budget to re-invent my diet, but I just need to be more mindful in my proportions and nutrients intake. He is right to say that dieting did not have to burn a hole in my pocket. Hence, thank you, Dr. Lau, for giving readers like me such valuable and sensible health insights."

— *Wendy Y.*

"Initially I was really dubious about Dr. Lau's scoliosis program, fearful of the fat in the diet. But I gave it a go. After about four weeks on the new diet, I started to really feel the benefits. My energy levels went up, the pain in my back disappeared, I now sleep all night without waking up, I no longer have cravings for chocolate or cheesecake, I feel great and I have lost 3kgs without even trying to lose it."

— *Isla W.*

"Backache had plagued me for more than 20 years. I thought it was due to bad posture or work-related. Acupuncture and massage only gave me temporary relief. I began my treatment with Dr. Kevin Lau 6 months after I had an X-ray taken. The results were beyond my expectation, 8 degrees in the thorax and 12 degrees in the lumbar and taller by 1cm."

— *Lucy K.*

"Dr. Lau is a kind-hearted man who understands the problems and pains suffered by his patients. He put his heart and soul in treating his patients. He shows concern and monitors the progress of his patients constantly. After Dr. Lau's program, I realized that my back problem and my health have improved. My overall conditions have improved. At long last, I have found someone who can help me in alleviating my back problem."

— *Christie C.*

"To me, the whole experience of the treatments meant much more than the 15 degrees of correction in my spine. I felt that in many ways I was blessed, and I learnt to have faith that there is a solution somewhere for any problem. Taking that on a very general estimate the scoliosis in an adult worsen by one degree per year, the corrections have perhaps saved me fifteen years... even if it is less, I am sincerely thankful for it."

— *Cher C.*

"Finally! I was independently healthy and pain free, the knowledge he offered me allowed me to sustain the health and wellbeing that I never thought I could have."

— *Alisa L.*

"Even more impressive is that Dr. Lau ordered my post therapy X-rays and it showed that I had reversed the degeneration in my spinal disc. I am so impressed with Dr. Lau's program. I admit to being skeptical at first, but the results I achieved have made me a believer! Thank you, Dr. Lau!"

— *Andre Z.*

HEALTH IN YOUR HANDS

Your Plan for Natural Scoliosis Prevention and Treatment

DR. KEVIN LAU D.C.

Dr Kevin Lau
302 Orchard Road #06-03,
Tong Building (Rolex Centre),
Singapore 238862.

For more information about the companion
Exercise DVD, Audiobook and ScolioTrack App for iPhone visit:

www.HIYH.info
or
www.Scoliosis.com.sg

Printed in the United States of America

ISBN: 1451568967
EAN-13: 9781451568967

Disclaimer

The information contained in this book is for educational purposes only. It is not intended to be used to diagnose or treat any disease, and is not a substitute or a prescription for proper medical advice, intervention, or treatment. Any consequences resulting from the application of this information will be the sole responsibility of the reader. Neither the authors nor the publishers will be liable for any damages caused, or alleged to be caused, by the application of the information in this book. Individuals with a known or suspected health condition are strongly encouraged to seek advice of a licensed healthcare professional before implementing any of the protocols in this book.

About the author

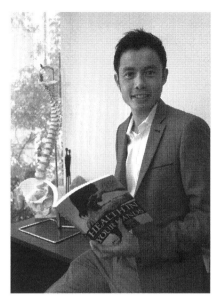

A graduate of RMIT University in Melbourne, Australia and Clayton College in Alabama, America, Dr. Kevin Lau D.C., combines university education with a lifetime of practicing natural and preventive medicine. His approach encompasses holistic treatment of body, mind and spirit.

After counseling hundreds of patients diagnosed with scoliosis and a host of other diseases, Dr. Lau discovered ground-breaking research that established, beyond a doubt, the clear merits of non-surgical treatment of scoliosis.

A firm believer in the ideology that health and sickness are within our control, Dr. Lau's main grounding has come from his own life experiences. His patients hail from all walks of life and have ranged in age from young children to ninety-year-olds. Dr. Lau was honored with the "Best Healthcare Provider Award" from the major newspaper publication in Singapore, Straits Time Newspaper.

Over the course of his career and based on his experiences, Dr. Lau has gained special expertise in treating patients with scoliosis, diabetes, depression, osteoarthritis, high blood pressure/hypertension, heart conditions, chronic neck and low back pain, and chronic tiredness, as well as several other "modern diseases".

Dr. Lau knows that the best medicine in the world comes straight from nature and it cannot be produced and mass marketed from a lab.

My Story

Growing up I lived a happy and healthy life, oblivious to the challenges that my health would later pose. When I turned 14, I started working in a fast food outlet where all that I subsisted on was burgers and chips on a regular basis. I drank gallons of sodas and milkshakes as if these were water, but no matter what I ate, I never put on an ounce of extra weight. I started noticing bad acne appearing on my face which made me painfully self-conscious, so I started trying every face wash product available, including scores of lotions and creams.

Later, when I moved interstate to study chiropractic, my health really began to deteriorate, going from bad to worse. At the age of 21, I became chronically ill and clinically depressed!

Away from my mother's cooking, I consumed instant ready-made meals and ate out of cans anything that could fill my stomach under a tight budget. I still remember going to the supermarket for the first time, ignoring the fruits and vegetables section and moving straight to the instant noodle, sugar-filled cereals and breakfast bars. As a consequence, gradually my skin began to worsen, but at the time I failed to connect the food and health together. Eventually my acne got so bad that I went to a medical doctor who immediately prescribed antibiotics.

The antibiotics did help initially, but I had to keep taking them, otherwise my skin would break out again. A few years of persistent dependence on antibiotics left me permanently scarred and riddled with digestive problems. I constantly felt haggard and tired, with the need to sleep all day. Intrinsically, I knew something was wrong with my system. My concentration and memory suffered; I went from a perfect "A" student to getting B's and, eventually, C's. Looking back on that period with the benefit of hindsight, I now understand that the majority of my problems were created by my naivety and a lack of understanding about the basic principles of nutrition. The antibiotics were merely treating the symptoms of acne and failed to treat the cause of which was due to poor diet.

Then something dramatic happened. One day, I "woke up," and gained true clarity. It marked a turning point in my life when I decided to go completely off all prescription medicine and started reading ferociously about natural health.

I read a lot of literature at this point and began to realize that practically everything that I had been doing up until then was leading up to one possible outcome - a slow poisoning of my normal, metabolic functioning. I had in effect turned into my own worst enemy. A thoughtless consumption of vast quantities of bad fats, sugar, pharmaceutical concoctions and the rigors of my study life, had begun to take their toll on my mind and body and were slowly leading me on a path of disease and depression.

You might call it a moment of reckoning. I was at a major crossroad of my life when I had just finished my studies and embarked upon my ultimate vocation: learning how to rebuild my body and regain my health bit by bit with consistent efforts and deliberation. I remember telling myself, how could I be practicing as a health professional if I wasn't a picture of good health?

From that point on I became a living example for my patients. Those that I attracted in droves were scoliosis patients because of modern medicines failure in effectively managing the condition. The results with these patients were at times so startling that I became convinced of my own methodology. Almost instinctively I knew I was on to something big; something that held the promise of health and hope to thousands of scoliosis patients around the world.

Today, as a practicing chiropractor and nutritionist, I am more certain than ever that scoliosis can be completely cured and treated. It may at one time have been one of the hardest and the most mysterious of all diseases, but today, with the application of the nutritional principles that I've incorporated, it can be completely arrested and the progress of the condition reversed. I've understood completely from my study of nutritional science that food alone has the miraculous healing properties to cure not only scoliosis, but a multitude of other diseases as well.

Over time, I've read practically every written word on traditional and alternative modes of healing. Some of this literature was inspiring and thoughtful; some contradicting and confusing. Nonetheless, since I was committed to total reformation, I began to make small but significant changes in my dietary and lifestyle patterns.

As my own patient, I started eating borderline vegetarian food and consuming 10 to 20 synthetic supplements a day, whilst drastically cutting out my sugar, processed foods and fat intake. I tried a host of things during this phase with mixed results, things as eccentric as spiritual healing to colonic therapy. I stuck to this routine for a few years in search of health truths.

Surprisingly for a major part of the day, although I still felt washed out, depressed and drained, I continued putting all my effort into my health, doing all the things that conventional knowledge said was bad, such as reducing fat, eating less meat and more vegetables. Yet I was not entirely happy with the progress (or lack thereof) that I was making. Things were not getting the momentum that I was hoping for.

After a meal, I still felt tired, mentally foggy and bloated. Digestive problems still plagued me to no ends to the point that food became my enemy. This was when I started a course in Masters in Holistic Nutrition and became inspired and hugely influenced by the work and writings of nutritional pioneers such as Dr. Weston Price, Dr. Joseph Mercola and Bill Wolcott. I admired other authors who were healed by nutritional therapies of incurable diseases where conventional drugs and surgery failed such as Gillian McKeith, TV presenter and author of "You Are What You Eat"; Mike Adams of NaturalNew.com and Jordan Rubin author of The Makers Diet.

Gradually, through their teachings, I learned to incorporate whole foods into my diet and started eating correctly for my Metabolic Type® and switched to consuming a lot of traditionally prepared probiotics like yogurt and kefir.

As I gained firmer knowledge of these fundamentals, I discovered that I was genetically "programmed" to be a protein type and that an over-emphasis on synthetic supplements was not helping. Indeed it was only making my health worse. By this time, I'd learned to read though the marketing hypes produced by food and supplement manufacturers and started to listen to my body.

I understood the importance of reducing grains and sugars from my diet and started to eat more protein and fat. Finally with all this and more, I understood the meaning of that well-known adage, "One person's food can be another person's poison."

Slowly but surely, with each new change that I introduced in my diet pattern, my health began to totter back to normal and started improving with each meal. No longer did eating make me feel tired, sleepy or foggy in the head. Instead, I started feeling extremely charged up and bursting with energy, calmness and mental clarity.

Emboldened by this experience, I finally decided to devote my life's work to exploring, gaining, and sharing more insights on nutrition, disease, health and healing with my patients, who trudged long distances to seek counsel with me.

In good health,

Dr. Kevin Lau

Acknowledgements

This book is dedicated to my family and patients, whose love, support, and inspiration helped me to piece together a better understanding of the workings of the spine and optimal health.

Additional Thanks And Credits

Nigel O'Brien (Graphic Designer, UK) - Who worked tireless on the front and back cover to make it stand out from the crowd.

Gisele Malenfant (Graphic Designer, Canada) - For designing the layout of the entire book and various inputs into making the book easier to read and general artistic direction.

Kathy Bruins (Editor, USA) - For her pervasive commitment to quality, and relentless attention to details.

Jacqueline Briggs (Illustrator, USA) - For the wonderful illustrations in the book and helping me to convey my ideas through the power of an image.

Darren Stephen Lim and Jason Chee (Personal Trainer, Singapore) - For demonstrating the exercises contained in this book and making it visually easier for readers to understand.

Photographer - Jericho Soh Chee Loon - For all the professionally taken exercise photos.

I would also like to thank the many dedicated scientists and clinicians whose own work inspired me, and contributed to my own.

Tips for Reading and Creating Your Own Scoliosis Correction Program

There is a lot of information packed into these pages! You'll be excited to find many answers to your scoliosis — but you'll probably be overwhelmed by all the things to know and do as you begin the program. Don't worry, things will fall into place when you follow the self assessments and step by step guide at the end of the book which is broken up into beginners and advanced.

I suggest reading the book all the way through, highlighting and jotting the ideas and actions you consider important. The empty column found at the side of each page is for these personal notes. Then, once you have completed the book and started on the diet and exercise program, go back and highlight in a different color, because you'll have a different point of view.

"A fool's talk brings a rod to
his back, but the lips of the wise
protect them."

— Proverbs 14:3

Table of Contents

Part 1 — What We Currently Know about Scoliosis

    1. The Future of Scoliosis Correction 21

    2. What is Scoliosis? 27

    3. Current Treatment Options for Scoliosis 43

    4. Shifting Away from Symptom-based Healthcare 59

    5. Ancient Bodies, Modern Diet 77

Part 2 — **A Nutritional Program for Health and Scoliosis**

    6. How is Nutrition Related to Scoliosis? 97

    7. Introduction to Fermented Foods 107

    8. Essential Carbohydrates 125

    9. Proteins the Bodies Building Blocks 137

    10. The Truth about Fats 145

    11. Nutrients for Bone and Joint Health 157

Part 3 — Corrective Exercises for Scoliosis

    12. How Your Spine Works...189

    13. Posture Retraining 205

    14. Body Balancing Stretches 213

    15. Building Your Core 239

    16. Body Alignment Exercises 259

    17. Living with Scoliosis 279

    18. Putting it All Together 305

    19. Readers Resource 313

Part 1

What We Currently Know about Scoliosis

CHAPTER 1

The Future of Scoliosis Correction

"Your life is in your hands, to make of it what you choose"

— *John Kehoe*

Ever since she could recall, Lucy Koh had suffered from chronic backache. She may have had it for almost 20 years. Now 54, Lucy thought her pain was work-related, perhaps caused by poor posture and a sedentary lifestyle. She met with dozens of acupuncture and massage experts. They gave her temporary relief, but the pain returned to torment her, as soon as she happened to discontinue with the program.

Gradually, as time wore on, her condition began to worsen and there were times when she felt a tingling sensation and acute numbness in her left arm and fingers. Alarmed, she finally sought consultation with an orthopedic surgeon.

After a few painful sessions of tractions and exercises with the therapist, a surgeon examined and discharged her saying her condition was probably caused by some kind of progressive muscular degeneration causing a nerve to get pinched. Beyond that, he could not identify the condition. He nonetheless suggested spinal surgery as a last resort.

Lucy understood the risks involved with surgery and refused the orthopedic doctors recommendation. She had more or less resigned herself to living with her pain, when one morning, she happened to glance at a public notice for a seminar presented by a chiropractor named Dr. Kevin Lau. More out of curiosity than conviction, she went to meet Dr. Lau.

He examined her and sent her for an X-ray. The report confirmed Dr. Lau's doubts. Lucy had scoliosis. Since this was the first time someone had at least diagnosed her condition correctly, a little skeptical at first, Lucy began her treatment with Dr. Lau. To begin with, she started attending his sessions each week and after six months, on Dr. Lau's suggestion got a second X-ray done.

The results? They were beyond her wildest expectations. Her scoliosis reduced by 8 degrees in the thorax and 12 degrees in the lumbar region and to crown it all, she was actually taller by 1cm as measured by her doctor during a routine check up at the hospital!

Expertly, Dr. Lau guided her through a detailed detoxification and individualized diet program. One year down the line, another series of tests were done and this time, as it turned out, Dr. Lau's treatment was not just improving Lucy's primary condition of scoliosis, but her diabetes, hypertension, cholesterol, kidneys and liver functions also improved with the changes proposed by Dr. Lau!

Meanwhile, Lucy's medical doctor prescribed a severe reduction in the amount of drugs she was taking and curtailed her earlier reliance on 12 different medications. Dr. Lau helped her identify the diet that is appropriate for her genetic/Metabolic Type® — protein type (you will learn more about that in this book) and prescribed an easy exercise regimen.

Needless to say, Lucy is extremely happy with the results. Friends compliment her and comment that she looks a picture of health. She also feels more energetic and doesn't tire of telling Dr. Lau that she feels she's entered a new phase in life.

Food as Medicine

As long as 2500 years ago, Hippocrates made this provocative statement: "Leave your drugs in the chemist's pot if you can heal the patient with food". Hippocrates recognized the importance of good nutrition to one's health, and took this concept a step further by trumpeting the healing properties of food.

Unfortunately, our modern culture has left this concept behind. Although scientists have made great strides in recognizing the elements that are present in our foods, and the diseases that are caused by a lack of certain nutrients in our diets, the idea of food as medicine became less popular in the modern world.

Consider the following: a person who eats processed, unhealthy foods all day long can be starving for nutrients, whereas someone who eats much less but chooses higher quality food will be in the peak of health. We have often heard the saying, "you are what you eat." This saying is truer than you know; eating unhealthy foods will eventually lead to poor health, while eating nutrient-rich foods will prevent many modern diseases. Everyone's nutritional requirements are different depending on their genetic makeup. Later in this book, you will learn how to eat for your right for your genes with Metabolic Typing®.

Eating the right foods in the right amounts is akin to taking preventative medicines and can help your body fight the effects of aging and other conditions caused by wearing down of the body. Eating the wrong foods, on the other hand, will lead to a buildup of toxins in your body, which will eventually overwhelm your natural defenses, causing illness.

Remember, an apple a day keeps the doctor away!

Healthcare: Past, Present and Future

Did you know that Egyptians consumed nothing stronger than cabbage to combat 87 deadly diseases; while onion was considered good enough to cure another 28! They of course didn't have an aspirin or Viagra in those days?

There has been research that proves that several conditions related to the diet of civilized societies are relatively absent from Aboriginal societies, helping them prevent many present-day degenerative diseases, dubbed as "lifestyle syndrome." Such diseases include: coronary heart diseases, high blood pressure, degenerated disc, osteoarthritis, appendicitis, gallstone, diabetes, obesity, strokes, hemorrhoids, hiatal hernia, dental caries, rectal polyps, varicose veins and cancers of the colon, ovaries and breast.

Fact: Modern society has seen a dramatic increase in killer diseases during the past 70 years

- Insanity increased 400%
- Cancer increased 308%
- Anemia increased 300%
- Epilepsy increased 397%
- Bright's Disease increased 65%
- Heart Disease increased 179%
- Diabetes increased 1800%
  (In spite of or because of insulin)
- Polio increased 680%

For instance, new research, published in the *New England Journal of Medicine* (2000; 343:16-22), has shown dramatic reductions in heart disease merely with the making of a few changes in the diet and general lifestyle of the patients. Another similar study proves that a few lifestyle changes can significantly stall the progress of prostate cancer, especially at early stages of detection in men.[1]

Is it any surprise then that the leading cause of death in our modern day society is not heart disease or cancer, but poor food habits?

In a study authored by Gary Null, Ph.D., Carolyn Dean, M.D., Martin Feldman, M.D., and others (2003), the authors agree that deaths caused by medicine can be put into a lengthy research report. According to these experts, nearly 751,936 Americans die every year as a result of medical error. In a manner, this is the equivalent of over six jumbo jets filled with passengers falling out of the sky every day!

Meanwhile, the number of people having in-hospital, adverse drug reactions (ADR) to prescribed medicine is around 2.2 million, while Dr. Richard Besser in 1995, revealed that the number of unnecessary antibiotics prescribed annually for viral infections was around 20 million!

A Point to Ponder On

"A successful practice of the healing art must be based upon the laws of life, the economy of vitality. The only foundation, therefore, of true healing is correct physiological principles; and here is precisely where the whole orthodox medical system of the present day fails — utterly and totally fails. It has no physiological and biological science upon which to truly practice the healing art."

— *R. T. Trall, M.D*

In 2003, this number increased to tens of millions of unnecessary antibiotics. Additionally around this time, the number of unnecessary medical and surgical procedures also increased to 7.5 million per year; while the number of people exposed to unnecessary hospitalization arose to 8.9 million. Small wonder that deaths caused by "medical errors" (the technical word is iatrogenic deaths) also rose to 783,936 during this interim.[2]

Let's face it: for nearly three decades, we have been hearing about the new dietary guidelines, miracle cures and wonder drugs. But the common problem with all these quick-fix options was that they were mass-oriented. They were not customized to the needs of a particular patient. Consequently, they invariably failed in their final or total impact.

Can you imagine a dress that would fit, say "all women aged 35, anywhere in the world?" Then how can you expect that of a medicine, which too must cater to a specific receiver? That's precisely the point that I've striven to make throughout this book.

In my understanding, scoliosis is merely a symptom of a deeper malaise; a bigger biochemical and mechanical dysfunction present in a person that appears as a disease. No two patients of scoliosis have the same bone density and no spine curvature is the same. So how can you expect that their treatment options to be the same? How can you expect that any standardized options (bracing or surgery) that has not been customized to their individual needs would produce equal gains?

It would not, as this book would set out to explain.

CHAPTER 2

What is Scoliosis?

When Susan was 12, her mother noticed a slight lump on her back. She immediately became concerned that it could be a tumor. The X-ray however, showed that her daughter's spine was growing sideways, curving in the shape of an S. The doctor said it was scoliosis.

Later X-rays revealed that Susan's spine was off-center 36 degrees. Her doctor said it was "idiopathic," which means that the cause is unknown. Approximately 80% of patients have this variety. The rest are usually attributed to birth defects, spinal cord injuries, and nerve and muscle diseases such as muscular dystrophy.

How is Scoliosis Detected?

What do Elizabeth Taylor, Sarah Michelle Gellar, Isabella Rossellini, and Vanessa Williams all have in common? Aside from the obvious fact that they are popular and gorgeous celebrities, these women all suffer from scoliosis. The disorder strikes two to three percent of all adolescents and generally becomes noticeable between the ages of 10 and 15, an age when an adolescent is very image-conscious. For unknown reasons, it affects more girls than boys - an inequality of about 3.6 to 1; and 10 to 1, when curves are 30 degrees or more. Symptoms typically include: one shoulder blade higher than the other, one hip raised, an uneven waist, the head not centered directly above the pelvis and leaning of the entire body to one side.

In 2008, it was found that 1 in 10 Singaporeans over 40 suffers from lumbar scoliosis, according to a study conducted by a team

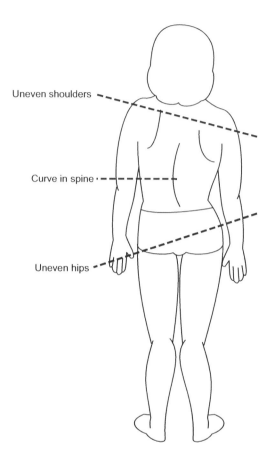

Uneven shoulders

Curve in spine

Uneven hips

Figure 1: Signs of Scoliosis

of spine surgeons. The study revealed that over 9% of those aged 40 and above have the condition. Worse, the study also revealed that the condition is 1.6 times more prevalent in women and that it occurred twice as often in Chinese and Malays than in Indians.[3]

Although the exact cause of scoliosis is still not known, doctors look for contributing factors in hormonal imbalances, poor nutrition, mechanical defect and genetic defects which have been linked to the disorder.

Finding Clues to the Cause of Scoliosis

Although doctors are still baffled by the medical riddle called scoliosis, they do know at least one thing, and that is what the nutritional causes of the conditions that tend to occur in conjunction with scoliosis. Some of the conditions that are known to appear concurrently with scoliosis are discussed below. An understanding of what causes these conditions would perhaps help us understand what causes scoliosis as well.

1. **Mitral valve prolapse (MVP)** - A heart disease that occurs frequently along with scoliosis. They may occur as "isolated" features, or together as common conditions found in many connective tissue disorders and other genetic disorders such as Down Syndrome.

    An Indian study found that 55% of the children with mitral valve prolapse had scoliosis.[4] Multiple studies have shown that in the majority of patients with mitral valve prolapse, as much as 85% are magnesium deficient and that magnesium supplementation alleviates the symptoms of MVP. Magnesium deficiencies have also been linked to osteoporosis and osteopenia, conditions also associated with scoliosis. With this many links, it would be logical to consider the possibility that a magnesium deficiency may be an underlying contributing factor in scoliosis.

    Magnesium deficiencies are also known to cause muscle contractions, and contracted muscles may play a role in scoliosis, as noted in another handful of posture studies on scoliosis.

    Interestingly, like idiopathic scoliosis, mitral valve prolapse is more common in females than males. Both mitral valve prolapse and idiopathic scoliosis appear to worsen at the beginning of puberty. Perhaps this is related to what Dr. Roger J. Williams has said about diet deficiencies that tend to occur during adolescence. Dr. Williams has pointed out in his books that the same diet that is perfectly adequate for young children may not be so for a child entering puberty, when nutritional requirements rise disproportionately to support sexual development.

It's also a well-documented fact that menstruating women are at greater risk of anemia than men due to the iron and magnesium lost during menstruation. However, these are not the only nutrients lost during menstruation.

2.   **Bleeding tendencies** - Multiple studies have demonstrated that Vitamin K deficits are also closely associated with both prolonged bleeding and osteoporosis, and are, perhaps, a contributory factor to the development of scoliosis.

Symptoms of prolonged bleeding caused by a vitamin K deficiency include hematuria (blood in the urine), easy bruising, heavy or prolonged menstrual bleeding, gastrointestinal bleeding, eye hemorrhages and nosebleeds.

3. **Hypoestrogenism (low estrogen levels)** - Low estrogen levels have long been linked to scoliosis in a variety of studies. The study of ballet dancers suggested that a delay in puberty along with prolonged intervals of menstruation reflect prolonged low levels of hypoestrogenism and may predispose ballet dancers[5] to scoliosis and stress fractures, where the incidence is 24—40%.[6] Low estrogen levels are a known cause of osteoporosis and osteopenia, conditions that many other studies have linked to scoliosis. Ballet dancers are thought to suffer from hypoestrogenism, because they tend to over-exercise and maintain low body weights, conditions that can cause low estrogen levels. In addition to ballet dancers, elite female athletes who train excessively also suffer from low estrogen levels, delayed

menarche, fractures and scoliosis. A 10-fold higher rate of scoliosis was found in rhythmic gymnastics trainees (12%) compared to a control group (1.1%).[7] Delay in menstruation and hypermobile joints are common in rhythmic gymnastics trainees.

Female athletes in general have high rates of scoliosis.[8] A likely reason for this is that women who exercise excessively, professional dancers and athletes, may stop menstruating, which in turn lowers their estrogen levels and puts them at risk for osteoporosis, a condition closely linked to scoliosis.

This increased risk of scoliosis and osteoporosis is similar to what happens when women reach menopause. Both athletes and post-menopausal women are at risk for low estrogen levels, fractures, osteopenia, scoliosis and osteoporosis. Perhaps it is because the low estrogen levels that occur in both groups of women cause weakened bones which result in osteoporosis, scoliosis and fractures.

Besides over-exercising and menopause, hypoestrogenism occurs along with scoliosis, caused by a host of nutritional deficiencies. These could include and not necessarily be limited to:

a) **Fractures** are linked to osteoporosis, which can be caused by a wide variety of nutritional deficiencies. A primary cause of both fractures and osteoporosis is a vitamin K deficiency. As noted above, vitamin K deficiencies can also cause bleeding tendencies, a condition which has also been linked to scoliosis.

b) **Hypermobility (double joints)** is a feature of rickets which has been linked to a wide variety of nutritional deficits, including deficits of vitamin D, calcium, magnesium (see mitral valve prolapse and magnesium above) and zinc.

c)   **Hypoestrogenism (delayed puberty & low body weights)** can be caused by deficiencies of zinc. Monkeys with zinc deficiencies have delayed sexual maturation, reduced weight gain and poor bone mineralization, many of the same conditions found in humans with scoliosis. Zinc deficiencies in humans have been linked to delayed puberty and low body weights. Zinc deficiencies in animal studies have likewise been shown to cause scoliosis.

4.   **Pectus excavatum (sunken chests)** - There is a statistically significant relationship between pectus excavatum and scoliosis. Pectus excavatum can be caused by rickets, which as noted above, can be caused by a wide variety of nutritional deficiencies.

Zinc deficiencies in monkeys have been known to cause a rachitic syndrome similar to rickets in humans. Interestingly, a separate study found gymnasts often had scoliosis and hypermobile joints, which are features of rickets.

Is It In Our Genes?

With the discovery of the human genome and the identification of the genetic causes of many diseases that resulted from this discovery, science has now moved beyond identification of risk factors for disease. The focus is now on what we can do to influence how our genes express themselves.

Our genes are what make us special and unique; they also help to determine what diseases or conditions we may be susceptible to. It was previously thought that we were "stuck" with the genes that we were handed, but scientists now have shown that we have more control over the expression of our genes than was previously thought.

There is much we can do to use our genes to our advantage, such as employing proper nutrition. Nutrients nourish our genes, and are even thought to turn our genes on and off. A good example of this can be demonstrated by cancer as a disease. It is known that cancer is often caused by cells multiplying at a far too rapid rate; this is how tumours form, which are basically growths caused by massive cellular proliferation. Nutrients may prevent these cells from being "turned on", thus preventing cancer. Nutrients work on many levels and in many ways throughout the body, and eating nutritiously may help you avoid developing cancer, even if you are genetically prone to certain types of cancer!

A new study led by scientists at the Medical Genetics Institute at Cedars-Sinai Medical Center has found that mutations of a certain gene lead to an inherited form of scoliosis.

The scientists indicated that the people who inherit this disorder, which is a type of a skeletal deformity, have a shorter-than-average trunk, limbs, fingers and toes. They are also affected by scoliosis, primarily in the lumbar vertebrae.

It is believed that mutations of the gene may cause increased calcium in the cells of the developing skeleton. While this is the first study to identify this mechanism as a contributor to this type of skeletal deformity, the findings suggest that calcium balance is important in normal spine development and hence the overall importance of nutrition in helping certain types of scoliosis even in those with a genetic predisposition.

Scoliosis Genetic Testing?

The ScoliScore AIS Prognostic Test is a new genetic test, which analyzes the DNA of patients who are diagnosed with Adolescent Idiopathic Scoliosis, the most common type of scoliosis. The test shows the likelihood of spinal curve progression. In other words, it helps doctors and patients to see how likely it is that a patient's spine will become more curved and whether it is likely that the patient will eventually need surgery or other interventions.

Approximately 85-90% of patients initially diagnosed with AIS will never have their mild (10-25° Cobb angle) scoliotic curve progress to a magnitude that requires surgical treatment. The test results may be used to predict, with over 99% probability, when a mild scoliotic curve is unlikely to progress to the point of requiring surgical treatment. This knowledge can prevent the need for these patients to undergo numerous office visits and exposure to radiographic imaging over many years to monitor potential curve progression.

What Scoliosis is NOT Caused By

I have been working with scoliosis patients for many years. The question I am asked most frequently is whether wrong sleeping position, poor posture, injury or carrying heavy objects causes scoliosis. The answer to this question is a resounding "no." Although these activities may cause pain or discomfort because they put strain on muscles and connective tissues, they do not, in and of themselves, cause scoliosis.

This is confirmed by other professionals who work closely with scoliosis patients, Dr. Arthur Steindler, of the University of Iowa, and Dr. Robert H. Lovett, orthopedists, noted poor posture as a cause for "false scoliosis," or a normal spine bent into a curved position. They did not believe poor posture or improper sitting, sleeping caused adolescent idiopathic scoliosis.

Scoliosis most commonly occurs during the adolescent growth spurt, and although there are many theories as to the cause of scoliosis, most cases are idiopathic, meaning that no obvious cause can be identified. It is likely that more than one factor contributes to the development of scoliosis.

Conclusion: So What Causes Scoliosis?

To summarize, many scoliosis researchers tend to spend a lot of time searching for a single cause of scoliosis. The common thread in many theories regarding the development and progression of scoliosis is some form of abnormality in either structural, neurological, biochemical or genetic makeup which leads to the wrong information regarding the body's orientation in space. My theory is that it is often the effect of multiple factors which leads to the development of scoliosis, such as a defective gene, abnormal biomechanical forces upon the spine, eating a poor diet leading to deficiencies or imbalances of nutrients, a physical asymmetry problem in the brain, and/or an imbalance in the hormonal system leading to a melatonin or estrogen deficiency.

By balancing our body chemistry through the foods that we are genetically meant to eat and the careful selection of an exercise program as detailed in this book, we can prevent and correct the symptoms of imbalance by educating the body on its correct orientation and alignment.

Scoliosis also tends to run in families, with recurrence among relatives reported at 25% and 35%.[9] When immediate family members such as parents and grandparents have scoliosis, the chance of developing scoliosis appears to be three or four times higher. When both parents are affected the number of children with significant curves was 40%, much higher than those without affected parents.[10] Since hereditary factors predispose a child to scoliosis, if someone in the family has scoliosis, you must be extra vigilant and be on the lookout for similar signs in other children. You must begin to radically amend your family's dietary habits, and incorporate a regular exercise routine as described in this book.

When is a Curve in the Spine Called Scoliosis?

Doctors generally don't worry about very mild spinal curvatures, i.e. anything below 10 degrees. These curves often straighten on their own, with only 3 in 1,000 worsening enough to need treatment.[11] However, when the curvature gets worse, the spine twists on its center, slowly pulling the rib cage out of normal position. Although most scoliosis curves are "S" shaped, some may even resemble a long "C."

Often, the first clue that scoliosis is developing is an uneven skirt hemline or a difference in pant-leg length. Other early warning signs, which often appear as poor posture to the untrained eye, include a hip or shoulder higher than the other, protruding shoulder blade, or tilted head.

It is known that curves greater than 30° are more likely to progress, having reached a point at which gravity has the advantage.[12] As a curve approaches 60 degrees, the distorted rib cage can restrict expansion of the lungs, causing breathing problems.

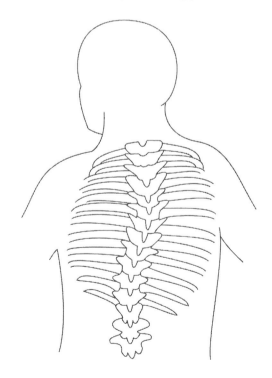

Figure 2: S-shape Scoliosis

Adams Forward Bend Test

The screening test used most often in schools and in the offices of pediatricians and primary care physicians is called the Adams Forward Bend Test.

The child bends forward dangling the arms, with the feet together and knees straight. The curve of structural scoliosis is more apparent when bending over. In a child with scoliosis, the examiner may observe an imbalanced rib cage, with one side being higher than the other, or other deformities.

The Adams Test, however, is not sensitive to abnormalities in the lower back, a very common site for scoliosis. Because the test misses about 15% of scoliosis cases, many experts do not recommend it as the sole method for screening for scoliosis.

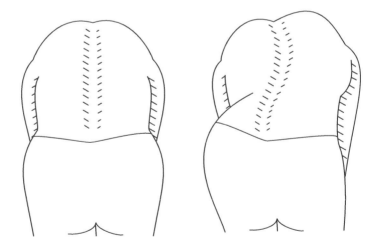

Figure 3: Adams test - normal spine (left), scoliotic spine (right)

Scoliosis Home Screen

Scoliosis can be accurately detected and monitored easily with the help of a family or friend in the comfort of their own home. You will need a pen and paper to record your answers. If you are concerned that your child may have scoliosis, follow these steps:

1) Using adhesive paper dots, place a dot on each of the bony prominences along the spine. This can be best accomplished by placing the dots on the bones of the spine that are visible to you. Once you have placed dots on the bones that you can see, you can run your fingers along the spine to feel the bones that are present but not visible. There should be 6 dots along the back of the neck (these may be easier to pinpoint if you ask your child to bend his/her neck), 12 dots down the mid-back, and 5 dots on the lower back. In all, you should have placed 23 dots, don't worry if you couldn't find them all.

2) With your child standing up straight but relaxed, and facing away from you, examine the row of dots to see if they form a straight line. Observe for the following from behind:

	NO	YES	
One shoulder is higher than the other	NO	Left	Right
Ribs are higher on one side than the other	NO	Left	Right
One shoulder blade protrudes more than the other	NO	Left	Right
One hip is higher than the other	NO	Left	Right
Lower back protrudes more on one side than the other side	NO	Left	Right

3) Ask your child to place their palms together and bend forward at the waist (Adams Test). Once again observe the following:

		YES	
Ribs are higher on one side than the other	NO	Left	Right
One shoulder blade protrudes more than the other	NO	Left	Right
One hip is higher than the other	NO	Left	Right
Lower back protrudes more on one side than the other side	NO	Left	Right

Results:

As you proceed through the steps, make note on Figure 4, which side an abnormality is on i.e. right shoulder appears higher when viewed from behind, ribs appear higher on the right when viewed from behind. If the line of dots that you have placed on your child's back appears to be crooked or uneven, make note of where the spine appears to curve on Figure 4. Is it in the lower back or upper back? Is there one or two curves? Also make note of the direction of the curve (right or left). Use the diagram on the next page to help map out your scoliosis:

If you answered yes to most of these observations then it should be brought to the attention of a health professional. A health professional, such as a family physician or chiropractor, will examine yourself or your child and be able to confirm whether or not it is scoliosis.

It is a good idea to perform this examination regularly during your child's adolescent growth spurts between 10 to 16 years of age, as this is when scoliosis is most commonly noted. Girls can

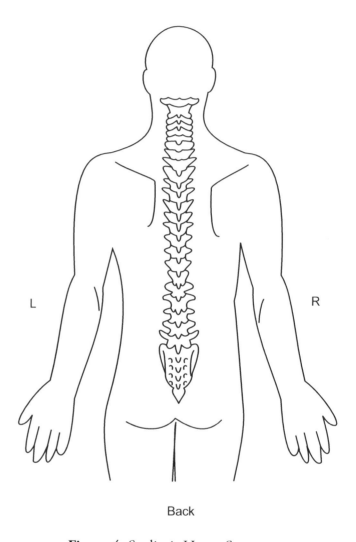

L   R

Back

Figure 4: Scoliosis Home Screen —
draw on the diagram your observations

wear a two-piece bathing suit to preserve modesty, while boys can
wear shorts. Scoliosis in children can be detected easily by parents
in the comfort of their own home. You will need a pen and paper
to record your answers or if following the methods described in
this book, I suggest taking a photo every 2 - 3 months to record
your progress.

How Scoliosis is Measured: The Cobb Angle

The most accurate method of determining the severity of a spinal curve is by taking measurements from an X-ray. Scoliosis is evaluated using the following criteria: the angle of the scoliosis, the side to which the curve deviates, the upper and lower vertebrae which form part of the curve and the apex vertebra, i.e., the vertebra which is furthest from the spinal midline. Evaluation of any spinal curvature detected on an X-ray film is usually done using the Cobb method. It involves identifying the curve, then finding the vertebrae at the top and bottom of the curve that have deviated the most from the horizon. When these

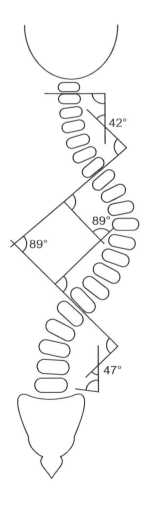

Figure 5: Cobbs Angle

two vertebrae have been identified, a straight horizontal line is drawn from the edges of both. The angle between these two lines is measured, and is given a numerical value, which is measured in degrees. This measurement is called the Cobb angle.

Although the Cobb angle is the standard for measuring spinal curvature, it has some drawbacks. For example, it cannot be determined if the spine has rotated (twisted) around the curve with this method, and therefore the severity of a curve may be underestimated when this method alone is used to measure a curve. However, the Cobbs angle is an excellent place to start, as full spine X-rays are easy and inexpensive to obtain.

Case Study: Scoliosis Correction at Any Age

Sixty-two year old Madam Chan had lived with scoliosis for most of her life symptom-free. Then one day while doing housework some 20 years ago, she bent down and felt a sharp pain in her spine. At the time, she did not consult any specialist to take care of the injury. There were times when it sent shooting pains up her spine that became so intense that it completely immobilized her for a few days, but as soon as it became better she forgot about it.

With her friend's persuasion, she later consulted a physiotherapist, which only helped to get rid of the pain temporarily. In 2003, she went for a hip replacement surgery. This gave her some relief, but the back problem persisted. In October 2005, she came to see me. Within a few months of therapy and working on her diet, her scoliosis and ultimately the pain it had caused had improved.

"At long last, I have found someone who can help me in alleviating my back problem."

— *Madam Chan (62 years old)*

CHAPTER 3

Current Treatment Options for Scoliosis

"If you limit your choices only to what seems possible or reasonable, you disconnect yourself from what you truly want, and all that is left is compromise."

— *Robert Fritz*

Decisions about conventional scoliosis treatment depend on the person's age, gender, general health, and potential for growth, as well as severity and location of the curve. Scoliosis affects 4.5% of the general population and scoliosis causes an average 14-year reduction in life expectancy.[13] Hence, preventing scoliosis in a pro-active way, as suggested by my diet and exercise regimen in this book, will add 168 million years of health and productivity to our society.[13] A closer look at the current treatment and management regimen will make it crystal clear why my regimen should be the preferred one for scoliosis patients. When it comes to scoliosis, medical doctors are notorious for recommending the wait-and-see approach. For a very mild curve medical doctors usually only advise monitoring checkups, with X-rays to detect worsening, every three or six months or maybe once a year. Even moderate curves of 25 to 40 degrees may not warrant treatment in their opinion other than bracing, but for a severe curve of 40 to 50 degrees, as a last resort they recommend spinal surgery. By then it's too late. The wait and see policy is synonymous to inviting problem by refusing to take action and is not based on rational thought process, but stems from a lack of treatment options from the surgeon to do anything useful. While surgery will always be an important treatment option for those with severe curvatures a lot more can been done in the early stages of their conditions to prevent it from getting worse.

Over the years, doctors have grappled very hard to understand what causes this abnormal curvature of the spine. It could be a result of an inability of a growing skeletal framework (vertebrae, discs, ligaments, ribs, pelvis, and lower limbs) to support itself during a time of growth spurt or be related to some neuromuscular dysfunction, connective tissue or genetic influences. The fact is that no single causal factor of scoliosis has been identified.

To Brace or Not to Brace?

There are several types of commonly used scoliosis braces:[14]

Thoraco-Lumbo-Sacral-Orthosis (TLSO)

The most common form of a TLSO brace is called the "Boston brace", and it may be referred to as an "underarm" brace. This brace is fitted to the child's body and custom molded from plastic. It works by applying three-point pressure to the curvature to prevent its progression. It can be worn under clothing and is typically not noticeable. The TLSO brace is usually worn 23 hours a day. This type of brace is usually prescribed for curves in the lumbar or thoraco-lumbar part of the spine.

Cervico-Thoraco-Lumbo-Sacral-Orthosis (known as a Milwaukee brace)

The Milwaukee brace is similar to the TLSO described above, but also includes a neck ring held in place by vertical bars attached to the body of the brace. It is also usually worn 23 hours a day. This type of brace is often prescribed for curves in the thoracic spine.

Charleston Bending Brace

This type of brace is also called a "nighttime" brace because it is only worn while sleeping. A Charleston back brace is molded to the patient while they are bent to the side, and thus applies more pressure and bends the child against the curve. This pressure improves the corrective action of the brace. This type of brace is worn only at night while the child is asleep. Curves must be in the 20 to 40 degree range and the apex of the curve needs to be below the level of the shoulder blade for the Charleston brace to be effective.

SpineCor Brace

The SpineCor is a newly discovered flexible brace system, usually prescribed in patients with a Cobb angle between 15° and 50°. Patients have to still wear it for at least 20 hours every day, until they have reached maturity, with radiological evaluations performed prior to and immediately following the fitting of the brace, and every 4 to 6 months afterwards. This bracing method incorporates a component to accommodate growth of the patient, whereby the components to the brace are expected to be changed every 1.5 to 2 years. A study conducted on juvenile idiopathic scoliosis patients termed the outcome of using the SpineCor brace as hugely successful.[15] But the Cochrane Library review classified this study as based on low quality evidence and also they did not find any subjective differences in the daily difficulties associated in wearing the SpineCor brace. It is important that such studies are performed based on guidelines for bracing studies of the Scoliosis Research Society (SRS) and the Society on Scoliosis Orthopedic and Rehabilitation Treatment (SOSORT) for the study outcome to be convincing.[16]

Effectiveness of Scoliosis Brace

As early as 1993, a report by the US Preventive Services Task Force noted that, "Beyond temporary correction of curves, there is inadequate evidence that braces limit the natural progression of the disease."[17] Then again, a 1984 study on scoliosis braces noted a "slight but insignificant" improvement in those who had been braced, "suggesting that bracing reduced the overall probability of progression in the braced curves." The study authors went on to report, "However, noting that nearly 75% of the control group curves were non-progressive, it is possible that a similar proportion of the braced curves need not have been braced."[18]

Years later, in 1995, a third study done by the Scoliosis Research Society found bracing to be effective.[19] However it is important to note that the study was sponsored by the Scoliosis Research Society, an industry body of orthopedists who could have had a definite monetary interest in continuing to prescribe bracing as a major treatment option for scoliosis. I personally think it is always prudent to view studies such as these, where the people funding the research stand to profit monetarily from the study findings, with a healthy dose of skepticism.

A 2007 study published in Spine by Drs. Dolan and Weinstein concluded that "observation only or scoliosis brace treatment showed no clear advantage of either approach.[20] Furthermore one can not recommend one approach over another to prevent scoliosis surgery. They gave the recommendation for bracing a grade "D" relative to observation only because of "troublingly inconsistent or inconclusive studies on any level." The rational way of gauging the effectivity of brace strategy will incorporate comparing results obtained in patients using brace against the expected genetic outcome of non-treated patients. Ogilvie et al. at Axial Bio-Tech performed a similar study and reported in 2009 in the journal Scoliosis that spinal brace has absolutely no positive effect on scoliosis.[21]

Research thus far has failed to prove definitively that bracing works, the investigators conclude. As reported by Dr. Stefano Negrini of the Italian Scientific Spine Institute of Milan, Italy, and colleagues report in The Cochrane Library (2010), the evidence for bracing is weak, as is the evidence of any long-term benefits of bracing. The available literature cumulatively constitutes "low quality evidence" in favor of using braces.[16] Questions and uncertainties about the effectiveness and need for use of brace for scoliosis will be more definitively answered once the five-year, multimillion-dollar study funded by the National Institute of Arthritis and Musculoskeletal and Skin Diseases results are analyzed impartially. The Spine Journal of September 2001 reported in an article titled 'Effectiveness of Bracing Male Patients with Idiopathic Scoliosis' that "Progression of 6 degrees occurred in 74% of boys and 46% reached surgical thresholds. Bracing of male patients with Idiopathic Scoliosis is ineffective."[22] In another article the 'Children's Research Center in Dublin, Ireland' states "Since 1991 bracing has not been recommended for children with AIS (Adolescent Idiopathic Scoliosis) at this center. It cannot be said to provide meaningful advantage to the patient or the community."[23]

On the other hand, Musculoskeletal Disorders reported a study on September 14th, 2004 titled, "Scoliosis treatment using a combination of manipulative and rehabilitative therapy," by Mark Morningstar, D.C., Dennis Woggon, D.C., and Gary Lawrence, D.C. 22 scoliosis patients with Cobb angles between 15 to 52 degrees were subjected to a rehabilitation protocol involving specific spinal adjustments, exercise therapy, and vibratory stimulation. Of the 19 patients completing the study, the average reduction in Cobb angle after 6 weeks was 62% (ranging between 8 to 33 degrees reduction and not even a single case of increase).[24] This warrants further expansion and testing of such innovative and non-invasive procedure that target the causes of scoliosis and not the manifested symptoms alone.

Despite all these studies, the standard non-surgical treatment for moderate curves (24 to 40 degrees) is still a body brace. Its non-cosmetic appearance is a major deterrent and the main reason for non-compliance, especially among girls. Conventional brace therapy carries several significant drawbacks. Because the brace stabilizes the spine by exerting pressure on the chest at critical points, it must envelop the trunk, and in so doing, can be bulky and uncomfortable. A brace also restricts body movement, which can over time cause atrophy and weakness of the chest and spinal musculature. As a result, the child's spine begins to lose some of its earlier flexibility and is prone to injury whenever the brace is taken off. When the muscles around the spine weaken, this can further complicate the scoliosis. Worse, in some cases the constant pressure of the brace can cause permanent deformation of the rib cage or the soft tissues directly under the pressure points.

In a recent study on the psychological impact of bracing on a growing child, it was revealed that "60% felt that bracing had handicapped their life and 14% considered that it had left a psychological scar."[25] Surely, you don't want any of those effects for your child?

Could Surgery Be An Option?

Obviously, if bracing was truly as effective as it is made out to be, then the need for spinal surgery would be reduced quite significantly. Unfortunately this is not the case. Of the 30,000 to 70,000 spinal surgery procedures done each year, about a third is performed for severe scoliosis.[26] While I believe surgery will always be a treatment option suitable for severe scoliosis, which is not conducive to other forms of treatments, I believe using the methods described in this book will surely help improve the health regardless of the severity of the curve. To help you make an informed choice about the treatment methods what follows is the different forms of scoliosis surgery as underlined below.[27, 28]

1. Harrington Procedure

This procedure was the most standard technique involved in scoliosis surgery until 10 years ago. The process involves use of a steel rod that extends from the bottom to the top of the curve, which in turn is supposed to support the fusion of the vertebrae. Pegs are inserted in the bones and serve as the anchors for the suspended rod(s). Of note, a full body cast and complete bed rest for 3-6 months is a pre-requisite post-surgery. Inexplicably, even though the rod is not required after 1-2 years, surgeons never think of taking out the rods until infection or other complications strike.

The standout disadvantages of the Harrington procedure are:

1. Extremely tough, especially for adolescents.

2. 10-25% loss of curve correction over time (which is 50% at best); additionally, the procedure is ineffective in correcting the spine rotation and hence does not alleviate the resultant rib hump.

3. Flat back syndrome in up to 40% of patients undergoing the procedure as it removes the normal inward curving of the lower back (lordosis). Prolonged duration of flat back syndrome might incapacitate a person by inhibiting a person to stand erect.

4. Chances of crankshaft phenomenon in kids younger than 11 years having the surgery. The underlying reason is continuing ossification process of the skeleton during the age of the surgery, and the front of the fused spine outgrows after the surgery. The spine curves as it cannot grow straight due to the traction.

2. Cotrel-Dubousset Procedure

Slightly better than Harrington procedure in that it remedial in principle for both the curve and the rotation of the spine, and flat back syndrome is not a complication. The procedure involves cross-linking parallel rods to render more stability to the fused vertebrae. The recovery time is around 3 weeks. The major disadvantages are the complexity of the surgery itself and the number of hooks and cross-links involved (Humke et al., 1995)[26].

3. The Texas Scottish-Rite Hospital (TSRH) Instrumentation

This is very similar in design to the Cotrel-Dubousset procedure, the only difference being use of smoother textured hooks and rods, which are supposed to make subsequent removal or readjustment in case of post-operative complications. Disadvantages also mimic the Cotrel-Dubousset protocol.

Other instrumentation that has been used is the Luque instrumentation,[29] which can maintain normal lordosis and was initially thought to circumvent the need of post-surgery brace use. But the flip side was curve correction achieved through surgery was completely reversed in the absence of brace usage and also resulted in incremental incidences of spinal cord injuries. Among others, Wisconsin Segmental Sine Instrumentation (WSSI)[30] is often used but seems to inherit the problems associated with the Luque as well as the Harrington rod procedures and is thus very problematic.

Surgeons have classically used the Posterior Approach[31] (access the surgical area through incision at the back of the patient), whereas Anterior Approach[32] (access the surgical area by opening the chest wall) finds lot of supporters among surgeons these days. The major complications arising out of the posterior approach are increased risk of occurrence of the crankshaft phenomenon, where the curve increases with time; and, not amicable to the thoracolumbar region. For the anterior approach, kyphosis (increasing outer curve), increased susceptibility to lung and chest infection, and pseudoarthrosis (pseudo joint at the fusion locale) are the major associated complications.

All this and more can be avoided simply by working on the health of the person through making some dietary changes and following an exercise routine, as described in this book. I've worked with hundreds of scoliosis patients and have come to the conclusion that often the cure does not lie in a one-stop surgery or uncomfortable bracing. Often, all that is needed is for the patient to be willing to take a proactive role in the improvement of their own health.

Food For Thought

"...The rate of surgeries performed in a given area has more to do with the number of surgeons in the area than the size of the population. One study showed that an area with 4.5 surgeons per 10,000 people experienced 940 operations per 10,000 while an area with 2.5 surgeons per 10,000 people experienced 590 operations per year."

— *Michael Murray,*
writing in Encyclopedia of Natural Medicine
and reporting on the 1989 paper by
L.L. Leape, "Unnecessay Surgery."

Examining the Risks of Spinal Surgery

Complications rate were estimated at 15% in children and 25% in adults for all fusion procedures in a study conducted between 1993 and 2002.[33] The major complications were as follows:

Blood Loss

Like for any surgical procedure there is significant blood loss which necessitates blood transfusion and so patients are encouraged to donate blood in the pre-operative period, causing further stress on the already suffering patient. Newer endoscopic techniques and use of recombinant human erythropoietin (rhEPO) to boost increased hematopoiesis are being examined to counter the blood loss.

Prone to infection

As with any other surgical procedure, chances of infection are pertinent in scoliosis surgery. Infection in the urinary tract and pancreas are most common and an antibiotic-coverage post-surgery is usually recommended.

Neuronal complications

Neuronal damage occurs in ~1% of patients undergoing surgery, with adults at a considerable higher risk than younger patients. Muscle weakness and/or paralysis are the usual outcome of nerve damage.

Pseudoarthrosis

Happens if the fusion does not heal and a pseudo joint develops at the site of surgery. It is a very painful condition. The anterior approach has higher chances of causing this complication, occurring upto in 20% of all surgery cases.

Low back pain and disk degeneration: The stress on the lower back as a result of the fusions in the lumbar region can ultimately result in disk degeneration. Additionally, compromised muscle strength, lower limb mobility, and balance can also cause excruciating back pain.

Pulmonary function

Younger adults and kids have high risk of developing pulmonary problems post-surgery upto about 2 months after the surgery. The risk is considerably higher in patients where scoliosis is a secondary outcome of neuromuscular problems.

Other than the above, gallstones, pancreatitis, intestinal obstruction and hardware injury (resulting from dislodged hooks, breakage of hooks and rusting, or a fracture in a fused vertebrae) are also associated with scoliosis surgery.

To alleviate some of the major concerns, few different forms (growing rod technique, vertebral body stapling and anterior spinal tethering) of minimally invasive surgery has been devised. Even though these techniques have shown short-term encouraging results, long term observance of effects and improvements are required for them to be considered seriously.

The Untold Truth about Scoliosis Surgery

The approximate average cost of scoliosis surgery in the U.S. is $120,000 per operation and there are roughly 20,000 such operation each year.[34] Shockingly, 8000 patients who had underwent scoliosis surgery become disabled each year, and in those who do not become disabled total recourse to the pre-operative condition happens within 22 years of surgery.[35] Additionally, there are follow-up surgeries to take care of loosened hooks, broken rods, rust formation![36] Worse, 25% of patients having surgery have compromised motor control post-surgery.[37] In some quarters it is suggested that the pitfalls of remedial surgery is actually worse than scoliosis itself. Are these not reasons enough to avoid surgery as the treatment regimen, until of course it is the last resort and pertinent? Do we not have a social responsibility to utilize and incorporate ways in our lifestyle that can significantly cut down on the critical and serious disadvantages of surgery? Precisely, my technique will lead you to just taking that first step towards your rehabilitation without even needing to resort to any of the dangers associated with scoliosis surgery. Alongside, it will improve your overall quality of life as understanding your disease and its cause is the beginning of the end of scoliosis in you.

Some true-life examples and case studies discussed here will reinforce my aforementioned assertions.

1. Stuart Weinstein, MD, University of Iowa reported in 2003 in the Journal of the American Medical Association (JAMA) "Many with curvature of spine go on to lead normal lives. Many adolescents diagnosed with spine curvatures can skip braces, surgery or other treatment without developing debilitating physical impairments, a 50 year study suggests."[38] ***Do we really need to incorporate bracing or surgery in young patients?***

2. Dr. J. Steinbeck reported in 2002 that "Forty percent of operated treated patients with idiopathic scoliosis were legally defined as severely handicapped persons 16.7 years after the surgery."[39] ***Does surgery really improve quality of life over time?***

3. Dr. Sponseller reported back in 1987 that "Frequency of pain was not reduced…pulmonary function did not change… 40% had minor complications, 20% had major complications, and… there was 1 death [out of 45 patients]. In view of the high rate of complications, the limited gains to be derived from spinal fusion should be assessed and clearly explained to the patient."[40] Why have we still persisted as surgery the method of choice?

4. Dr. H Moriya reported in 2005 that "Corrosion was seen on many of the rod junctions (66.2%) after long-term implantation."[41]

Why are effective and less dangerous alternatives not being embraced?

5. Reuters Health (New York) reported on Jan 29, 2008: "Screening for scoliosis and subsequent brace treatment appears to be of no utility in avoiding surgery, Dutch researchers report in the January issue of Pediatrics for Parents. "We think that abolishing screening for scoliosis seems justified," lead investigator Eveline M. Bunge told Reuters Health. This is "because of the lack of evidence that screening and/or early treatment by bracing is beneficial."[42]

6. Dr. M. Hawes reported in The Journal of Pediatric Rehabilitation that "Pediatric scoliosis is associated with signs and symptoms including reduced pulmonary function, increased pain and impaired quality of life, all of which worsen during adulthood, even when the curvature remains stable. In 1941, the American Orthopedic Association reported that for 70% of patients treated surgically, the outcome was fair or poor.... Successful surgery still does not eliminate spinal curvature and it introduces irreversible complications whose long-term impact is poorly understood. For most patients there is little or no improvement in pulmonary function.... The rib deformity is eliminated only by rib resection which can dramatically reduce respiratory function even in healthy adolescents. Outcome for pulmonary function and deformity is worse in patients treated surgically before the age of 10 years, despite earlier intervention. Research to develop effective non-surgical methods to prevent progression of mild, reversible spinal curvatures into complex, irreversible spinal deformities is long overdue."[43] ***Do we really need surgery?***

Why the Methods in this Book is Better

Hereditary pre-disposition: James W. Ogilvie's group discovered genetic markers, two major genetic loci and 12 minor loci that are related to the development of scoliosis. 95% of patients having a curve greater than 40 degrees had a correlation to the identified genetic markers.[44] Hence, it is now possible to predict the hereditary predisposition to scoliosis and based on the same, individualized management regimen can be laid out using my comprehensive care therapeutic strategy, which has the added advantage of being completely non-invasive. The main reason for all these procedures not working is that they try to cure the condition and not the cause. While we are powerless to change our genes we can still change the way it interacts with the environment and thus suppress these genetic faults and how they are ultimately expressed through disease. This is where my proposed regimen of balancing metabolic, neurological and biochemical homeostatic factors using of customized nutrition, exercises and lifestyle regime will be most effective-weed out the cause of scoliosis.

Claire's Personal Story

Like most young girls, Claire C. didn't know about scoliosis until she was diagnosed with it during her secondary school scoliosis screen. At that time, it was only 15 degrees and was told to come back in 6 months for another review. When 6 months had passed, the doctor requested an X-ray, which revealed her scoliosis had progressed. Claire was suffering from a primary low back curvature of almost 40 degrees and a smaller compensatory thoracic (mid to upper back) curvature of about 34 degrees.

She wasn't suffering from any pain yet, but she did have a noticeable hump on her back and uneven shoulders which concerned her parents. With the advice of her orthopaedic doctor she was immediately fitted with a hard brace and was told if her curve progressed any further she would need scoliosis surgery.

She was told to wear the brace for 23 hours daily in the hope to prevent her spine from getting any worse. But in the hot, humid climate of Singapore, the brace was extremely uncomfortable, and after about a month, Claire couldn't take the pain and irritation from the brace any longer and stopped wearing it.

Claire and her family began to look for alternative treatments, fearing that a high-risk surgery was all that current prescribed medicine could offer her. That's when they found Dr. Kevin, and in six months of treatment, her scoliosis had been reduced by 28 degrees! Her shoulder imbalance and the hump on her back had noticeably improved.

She returned to the orthopaedic specialist for a follow up, and he was amazed at her improvement. He immediately attributed the success to the brace; the one she had stopped wearing!

Because of her refusal to accept one answer for treating her scoliosis, Claire was able to avoid bracing and a risky surgery.

> "Bracing was not effective at all. I was not able to use it as recommended as it was extremely uncomfortable and inconvenient; as such, I gave up wearing it after some time. Surgery on the other hand wasn't any better. I was afraid of the complications and the pain and the scar it left. With Dr Kevin's program I was able to avoid them both!"
>
> — *Claire C. (16 years old)*

CHAPTER 4

Shifting Away from Symptom-based Healthcare

"Unfortunately, everything the experts tell us about diet is aimed at the whole population, and we are not all the same."

— *The Scientist magazine*

Tell me: how many times have you consulted a medical doctor who did not claim to have a ready remedy (a drug) for every disease?

The common refrain is: if you suffer from this, try this. If you suffer from that, try that. In the end, the list of drugs prescribed could be longer than the number of identified diseases in the world!

I've learned that this is just a ruse. Allopathic preparations or drugs don't cure; they only mask the symptoms. The body is the only thing that cures the disease, but only if you allow it to. Drugs merely eliminate the symptoms of a disease and you begin to feel better for it because, after all, symptoms are what bother you. Drugs don't usually get to the bottom of the problem. That's the reason they don't offer a permanent cure. They just ensure life-time customers for the pharmacist and the drug manufacturers.

To cite an example, imagine you are driving a car and spot a flashing red light on your dashboard that turns on. This is the symptom. This light tells you that the car is overheating, in this case due to a leak from the cooling system. This is the cause.

You take your car to a mechanic (the medical doctor), and he cuts the wire that turns the light on, and tells you the problem is solved. You are fine for now. He tells you to put water in the cooling system every day and add oil when needed and buy these things from any pharmacy. This is treating the symptom and hooking you to consume the medication, in this case water and oil, forever. They force you to buy from them. You can never drive that car without those medications and one day, your trustworthy old car will simply conk out.

The problem with this kind of an approach is you never get to fix the leak.

Our industrial society has established a new image of the human body. Patients have begun to believe that their bodies are repairable machines that can be diagnosed, measured, monitored, and kept alive by other machines. This new body image is even reflected in our lexicon: "nervous breakdown," "blow off steam," "recharge your batteries," or "reprogram myself." Some patients, as a result, regard their doctors as mechanics, plumbers, electricians, or carpenters, rather than healers.

Physicians also tend to diagnose and treat patients based on a model of health or disease to which that particular patient may or may not culturally subscribe to. Many people dissatisfied with the purely biological view of illness are now seeking alternative, holistic treatments.

As a chiropractor and nutritionist specializing in the care of patients with scoliosis, I have always believed in our body's innate ability to heal and regenerate. A medical doctor would promise symptomatic relief in the form of surgery and bracing; I would treat fundamental imbalance present in the body with food and recommend appropriate exercise and physical therapy to correct the deformity.

My advice to my patients often is: don't follow any fads or marketing hypes. Listen to your body's unique needs and give your body just what it demands. Your body has the innate wisdom to regulate all complex functions and restore healthy equilibrium. This book will teach you how to pay heed to this expert's advice.

Nutrition Fact: One Size Does Not Fit All

Did you as a child, ever happen to participate in a tug-of-war, where one side pulls one end of a long rope and the other the opposite end, in order to see who would eventually be able to pull the longest length of the rope? The rope generally broke in two with all this pulling.

In my mind, in this great diet debate, we are witnessing something similar: a nutritional tug-of-war. For a while, the general consensus would be that a high protein, low carbohydrate diet was the best for health and weight loss. After a period of time high carbohydrates were in fashion, but high protein diets were out. Each dietary ideology had its devoted advocates and followers who had success with a particular diet, yet the number of failures was the same. Things have come to such a pass that these days everybody is confused - should I follow this diet or that?

For instance, I've known patients who have tried at least six different fad diets before they end up in my clinic and by that time they are totally exhausted and morally discouraged, because the various diets have also wrought havoc with their systems and produced results that were often counterproductive!

Don't let that happen to you. In my opinion, these experts have turned out to be wrong; dead wrong for some and seriously wrong for millions of others. Instead of fulfilling their promise, this latest "right diet for all people," they have unwittingly given rise to mass confusion of what is considered healthy, and obesity of the kind that modern societies have never seen before, along with the "bonus" side-effect of an ever-increasing number of diabetics.

During my early days of practice, dietary recommendations were often a hit or a miss affair. I would design a "healthy" diet that would work for a group of patients, but for many others they simply didn't help. Indeed, in some cases, it even made their condition worse!

I was so frustrated that even with the lack of consistency in the results that I was getting, I still felt motivated to further my research into nutrition. It was at this point that I happened to read a book by William Wolcott. His concept of Metabolic Typing® completely revolutionized my thinking and suddenly all the missing pieces of the jigsaw puzzle began to fall into place. I realized then that each one of us is different from the other; so our nutrient requirement from the food that we consume is also different.

Just think: We all look different on the outside and we also function differently on the inside, so why should we all eat the same diet? I would call this junk nutritional science!

Dietary Evolution

I once came across a very brilliant, thought-provoking piece by the University of Utah's famous anthropologist, Henry Harpending.

In that piece published as a report in *Science Daily*,[45] the author wrote, "We aren't the same as people even 1,000 or 2,000 years ago and the reason that he cites for this is a strong genetic influence." He mentions that researchers have discovered genetic evidence that human evolution is speeding up — and has not halted or proceeded at a constant rate, as was imagined before, thus indicating that human beings on different continents are increasingly becoming different.

Indeed, Harpending's study shows that humans are changing relatively rapidly on a scale of centuries to millennia, and that these changes are different among different continental groups. Interestingly, this study backs up a similar conclusion that a Harvard-trained dentist, Dr. Weston A. Price, arrived at several years ago. (*You will read more about it in our next chapter*).

Harpending mentions that rapid population growth has been coupled with vast changes in cultures and environment, creating new opportunities for adaptation.

"The past 10,000 years have seen rapid skeletal and dental evolution in human populations, as well as the appearance of many new genetic responses to diet and disease," he writes.

The issue is that we as a race have not kept pace with the evolutionary changes and the resulting changes in our dietary patterns. Harpending's research notes that human migrations into new Eurasian environments created selective pressures favoring less skin pigmentation (so more sunlight could be absorbed by skin to make vitamin D), adaptation to cold weather and certain dietary changes.

Because the human population grew from several million at the end of the Ice Age to 6 billion in the present day, more favored new genes have emerged and evolution has speeded up, both globally and among continental groups of people, Harpending says.

For example, in China and most of Africa, few people can digest fresh milk into adulthood. Yet in Sweden and Denmark, the gene that makes the milk-digesting enzyme lactase remains active, so almost everyone can drink fresh milk," explaining why milk is more common in Europe than in Asia and Africa.

"If you suddenly take hunter-gatherers and give them a diet of corn, rice or wheat, they frequently get diabetes. We're still adapting to that. Several new genes we see spreading through the population are involved with helping us prosper with high-carbohydrate diet," says Harpending.

Case Study: Low Back Pain, High Cholesterol and Digestive Problems

Before she met me, Alisa L. (56, School Teacher) suffered from severe lower back ache, high cholesterol and massive digestive problems. She had consulted various doctors, specialists and massage therapists only to have her issues reoccur whenever she stopped the treatment. Alisa L. was a classic "hunter and gather" living in a modern society filled with sugars and grains. After teaching her the foods which helped to balance her body and eliminating those that lead to poor health, her back pain, high cholesterol and digestive problems improved.

From a letter she wrote to me after her treatments with me,

> "…thank you to Dr.Kevin who has a caring heart and listening ear. He is an inspiration to all other patients. His holistic approach to health was what I needed. I made and stuck to the right lifestyle, eating habits and mental attitude and fought for my health. My low back pain and digestive issues disappeared and my cholesterol is back to normal. Finally, I'm in control of my health, drug free and pain free. What's more, others have commented that I even look younger."

> — *Alisa L. (56 years old)*

The Future of Nutritional Science

Tell me: Can you fill your car with diesel when it's designed for gasoline?

Will it *ever* run smoothly?

I would assert that the same goes for your body. The food that you supply it with can either make it run efficiently (like your car) so that it contributes to meeting your genetic requirements or, if you happen to put the wrong fuel inside it, you begin to feel all the negative effects, such as feeling tired, inefficient and "not well," all of which can actually accentuate your genetic flaws.

In any case, the concept of recommending different diets for different people is nothing new. Ancient Greeks and Romans made that famous proclamation "one man's food is another man's poison."

Likewise, in the Far East, Chinese medicine has taught us that we are all born with a different constitution and therefore require different kinds of food based on our unique characteristics and energetic imbalances. The 5,000 year old Ayurvedic medicine of India in fact has identified three main body types and diseases (*dorshas*): *pitta, vatta* and *kapha* — each with its own specific dietary needs and problem areas.

The author of the book, William Wolcott, and other modern nutritional researchers came to the same conclusion, that there are three metabolic "types": protein; carbohydrate and mixed types. What we need for optimal health has so much to do with our genetic coding and our cultural background.

People who are protein types must concentrate on high-density, high "purine" proteins available in dark meats such as chicken thighs, lamb, beef and salmon, including the organs. They must limit their intake of high glycemic carbohydrate foods such as sugars, refined grains and potatoes. Instead, they must focus on whole grains and low glycemic vegetables such as asparagus, fresh green beans, cauliflower, spinach, celery and mushrooms. They must limit the amount of fruit they consume because protein types tend to develop blood sugar problems; coconut, avocados, black and green olives, green apples and pears are their best choices. They must also snack more often and avoid alcohol in any form.

On the other side of the spectrum, the carbohydrate type must concentrate on low protein (low purine), low fat sources such as chicken and fish and vegetables. These individuals also do very well on starch. While their bodies are better able to tolerate high starch food like legumes and grains they should still eat these foods in moderation. All fruits are fine, but berries and citrus fruits are particularly good.

In the reader's resource section, you will find a shopping list that you can tailor to your food requirements appropriate to your Metabolic Type®. The easiest way to estimating the proportions of food you need is to visualize a plate and then covering it with the correct percentage of each food type as shown in Figure 6: Meal Proportions.

At its most fundamental level, Metabolic Typing® places you into one of three categories:

1. **Protein Types**
2. **Mixed types**
3. **Carbohydrate Types**

These basic types speak volumes about the way your body functions on an internal plane and the way your system processes food and absorbs nutrients. There are anatomical differences and physical evidence that show that the basic form and shape of our stomachs also differs vastly from one another.

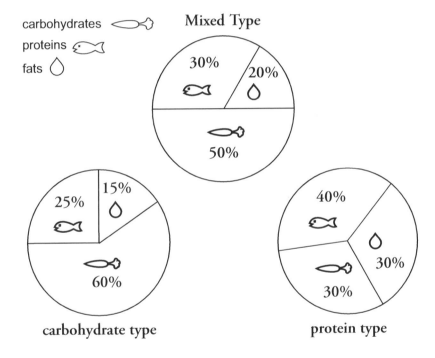

Figure 6: Meal Proportions

The fact is that although we all need a full spectrum of nutrients, different people need these nutrients in different doses. It is these different genetic-based requirements that explain why a certain nutrient can cause one person to feel good, have no effect on another; and cause a third person to feel worse.

Thus the biggest myth that Metabolic Typing® demolishes is that there are universal dietary fixes for human beings. This mass market approach to nutrition in fact does more harm than good. While recommending a universal formula for everyone, it fails to take into account exactly how much protein, carbohydrates or fats people should be consuming and in exactly what proportion. Even if they are able to record some initial progress it's because they are playing a game of dietary roulette: sometimes they hit the jackpot, but most often they fail.

Indeed, if life were as simple as some of these self-proclaimed gurus of modern diets make it out to be, there wouldn't be so much disease in this world, or would there?

The bottom line is that dietary nutrients must be tailored to individual needs, because what works best for one person may be poison for another. My hope is that this is really the beginning of personalized medicine for the masses. It's crazy the way our health-care system has treated us all like we're one and the same person. We're all completely unique. We respond differently to diet, and we respond differently to medications and some small part of that, some people say as much as 20 percent—can be linked to our genetic differences.

However, not every difference can be attributed to genetics. Some of these differences are also caused by environmental factors. For instance, people who inhabit tropical regions have strong hereditary needs for diets high in carbohydrates, such as vegetables, fruits, grains and legumes. This is the kind of "biofuel" their body needs to keep the machine running and in good condition. They are indeed genetically programmed to process just this kind of food.

In sharp contrast, Eskimos can easily consume up to 90% quantities of fat and proteins from seals and whales because that's exactly what their body demands to weather the extreme cold conditions of their habitat. Interestingly they are also relatively free of heart disease despite a high-fat, high-cholesterol diet.

Therefore, a diet considered healthy in one part of the world may be all wrong and potentially poisonous for people living in another part of the world.

Making a similar point, Dr. Lendon Smith writes in his book *Happiness Is a Healthy Life*, "The trick of eating is to figure out your racial/ethnic background and try to imitate it." However, as moving from one continent to another has become as easy as buying a plane ticket online, we might have parents from different racial backgrounds and we cannot base our dietary habits simply on where we are from.

This is where Metabolic Typing® comes in handy. It helps you find the perfect balance of food macronutrients — protein, carbohydrates and fats that your body needs based on our own bodies reactions to food.

In the past, we lacked the clinical knowledge to enable us to understand why we have the diseases we do. But today, thanks largely to the work done by Dr. Price, Dr. Williams and other researchers, we can determine the correct nutritional requirement of each person on a case-by-case basis. It is a different matter altogether that a given metabolic imbalance can manifest in a variety of ways, in the form of a number of different diseases or degenerative processes.

In 1956, Dr. Roger Williams wrote a revolutionary book titled *Biochemical Individuality*, in which he posited that individuality pervades every nook and crevice of our body, that human beings are highly distinctive on a microscopic cellular level and that these inherited differences extend to our basic structure and metabolic processing as well. Therefore, imbalances or inadequate nutrients at the cellular level could be the one major root cause of any disease. These findings were so startling that Dr. Williams quickly became one of the earliest proponents of Metabolic Typing®.

The Metabolic Type® model that we are going to discuss in this book is more accurate as you listen to your own body for clues on what foods would help to restore it to balance and correct the disorders, naturally. In my observation, people who faithfully follow the Metabolic Typing® model discussed here register great improvement in their body and mind within a short span of time, sometimes as soon as one month. Can it get any better than that?

Unfortunately, much of what our culture promotes as a medical system is based on treating symptoms and not addressing the underlying cause of those symptoms. Therefore, conventional medicine really has a limited ability to resolve most of the chronic illnesses that we suffer from today, although they may be effective for some acute health challenges. If we begin to resolve personal biochemical imbalances that are the underlying causes of disease through the model that I recommend in this book, you will have the unique ability to balance your total body chemistry and ensure proper growth of the body and spine.

Addressing disease processes such as scoliosis at their causative, root level before they turn chronic can:

- Ensure proper growth of your body
- Prevent illness in terms of several opportunistic diseases
- Rebuild your immunological response system, so you don't catch infection easily
- Provide you with uniquely long-lasting health benefits

In short, when you begin eating correctly for your Metabolic Type®, your body system will gradually begin to veer towards total balance; a balance of spirit, mind and body. As you do this, your body will produce energy more efficiently from foods that you consume to make you heal and grow healthier.

When you are metabolically balanced, you will naturally have more energy at your command than you ever thought possible before. You will have created an inner cellular environment that is conducive to experiencing your highest levels of:

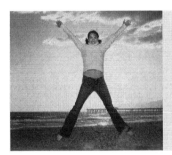

- Peaceful energy
- Relaxed alertness
- Emotional poise
- Positive stable mood
- Great mental clarity

When you eat the foods that your body is not designed to eat, it will protest. This protest will appear as symptoms of a disease, with the result that you may feel bloated, tired, and constantly hungry or feel irrational food cravings even after a full meal!

Does this sound familiar? Here, I go back to my previous point: when our genetic make-up, our personalities and our facial features are so dissimilar, why would our nutritional needs be similar? My goal is to help you become more attuned to what your body needs from one meal to the next to optimize your genetic potential and suppress the genetic weaknesses that create disease.

Simultaneously, it should be acknowledged that while there could be a genetic predisposition to chronic diseases such as scoliosis, diabetes and obesity—and, in all likelihood, to many other illnesses as well—in almost all cases, it is just a predisposition, not the pronouncement of a death sentence. Therefore, even if your mother or father or sister had scoliosis, it doesn't mean that you will have it too. All that it implies is that you will have a greater genetic predisposition to it and, therefore, will need to make bigger changes in your diet and lifestyle than someone born with an altogether different set of genes. In any case, a foreknowledge of these genetic limitations is a good thing. It helps you prepare against all potential ailments that may strike you later in life. It can make you more proactive in choosing the right lifestyle for yourself.

What about the Blood Type Diet?

The Blood Type diet, proposed by Peter D'Adamo, N.D., and popularized in his book *Eat Right for Your Type* (Putman, 1997) was indeed a precursor to the more sophisticated Metabolic Type® diet that evolved later. The Blood Type diet, as the name itself indicates, is based on the premise that our nutritional needs are determined by our blood type classification, i.e., O, A, B or AB.

However, this was an oversimplification of a more complex picture. With ethnic group migration and more diversity entering into our midst, none of us can really be sure of our genetic heritage. If a Chinese and a person of European descent both have the blood type "O", should they be eating the same types of foods? What of the person who is Eurasian? Won't this mixed heritage further confuse the issue? How about a person going through different stages of life such as puberty, pregnancy or menopause? Wouldn't their nutritional need be different at different phases?

This is where Metabolic Typing® can be very useful. A major goal of this model is to determine which foods and what amounts are best for your particular type and no other. It focuses on customizing a person's diet based on his/her individual needs and reactions to foods, regardless of the person's blood types or any other sweeping generalizations.

Metabolic Typing Challenge

If you don't believe that there could be any such thing as metabolic individuality and if you don't believe that everyone can be healthy and at his peak performance by eating just any kind of diet, here is the Metabolic Typing® Challenge.

Follow the instructions very carefully. Then have your spouse, your children, and your friends take it as well. Compare the results. You may be amazed to find out how different we can be from one another, even within the same family. ***Now realize that these differences also relate to which foods are good for us and which are not.*** If there really is one diet that is right for everyone, why are there hundreds of diets on the market and more and more each year? Why does one diet make one person slimmer and another one fatter? The only solution is to find out what's right for YOUR body not your spouse's or your friend's, but what is right for YOU!

- Place a check mark to the left of each answer that BEST APPLIES to you
- Choose only one answer per query
- If no answer applies to you, leave that query unchecked/ unanswered

IMPORTANT: The choices as written may not describe you exactly. So, it is VERY IMPORTANT that you choose the answer that best describes your TENDENCIES. The provided answer need not be a perfect description, just an indication of your trend in that direction. If you definitely fall somewhere in between, skip that query and go on to the next one.

Metabolic Typing Challenge

✔	ANSWER #1	***DIET QUERY***	✔	ANSWER #2
	Tend toward weak, lacking, or diminished	APPETITE (In general)		Tend towards strong, voracious, ravenous
	Love sweets, often need something sweet with meal to feel satisfied	DESSERTS		Don't really care for sweets desserts, but may like something fatty or salty (like cheese, chips or popcorn) for a snack after meals
	Usually worsens sleep, especially if heavy food	EATING BEFORE BED		Usually improves sleep
	"Eat to live" — unconcerned with food and eating	EATING HABITS		"Live to eat" — need to eat often to feel good, be at best
	Doesn't bother	4 HOURS+WITHOUT EATING		Makes irritable, jittery, weak, famished or depressed
	Energizes, satisfies me	ORANGE JUICE ALONE		Can make me light-headed, hungry, jittery, shaky, or nauseated
	Can skip with no ill effects	SKIPPING MEALS		Must eat regularly (OR OFTEN); don't do well if I skip a meal
	Rarely or never want snacks and/ or prefer something sweet when I do	SNACKING		Often want to eat between meals and/prefer something salty or fatty
		DIET SECTION TOTALS		

✔	ANSWER #1	***PHYSICAL QUERY***	✔	ANSWER #2
	Taller, leaner	BUILD		Shorter, thicker
	Belching, burping, gas, full feeling after meals, slow digestion, careful what eat	DIGESTION What is your tendency?		Easily digest most foods, rapid digestion, no real digestive complains
	Pale , light	EAR COLOUR		Flushed ,pink ,rosy
	Larger than iris in average lighted room	EYES — PUPIL SIZE [Pupils black, center portion of eyes. Iris = coloured part of eyes]		Smaller than iris in average lighted room
	Cool , cold	HANDS - TEMPERATURE		Warm
	Bothersome , need sunglasses	LIGHT — STRONG , BRIGHT		Doesn't really bother
	Tend toward dull , unclear	SKIN — FACIAL COMPLEXION		Tend toward bright , clear
	Mild reaction , go quickly	SKIN — INSECT BITES/STINGS		Strong reaction , go away quickly
		PHYSICAL SECTION TOTALS		

✔	ANSWER #1	***PSYCH QUERY***	✔	ANSWER #2
	Overachiever (Type A Personality)	ACHIEVEMENT		Underachiever (Type B Personality)
	Very active, find it hard to slow down, tend toward hyperactivity	ACTIVITY LEVEL		Not real active, prefer to be more sedentary, find it easy to be inactive
	Quick to anger, emotional outbursts	ANGER		Slow to anger. More even - tempered
	Early to bed, early to rise	ARISING/RETIRING TIME (natural, without alarm clock)		Late to bed, late to rise
	Love/prefer/do best in warm or hot weather	CLIMATE PREFERENCE		Do better, feel invigorated in cold weather, do poorly in warm/hot weather
	Tend to be	COMPETITIVE		Tend not to be
	Poor	ENDURANCE		Good
	Easy to put thoughts into words	EXPRESSION OF THOUGHT		Hard to put thoughts into words
	Love it	EXERCISE		Don't care for it
	Tend to be	IMPATIENT		Rarely, tend to be patient
	Very organized	ORGANIZATION		Tend to be disorganized, take things as they come
	Perfectionist	PERFECTION		Not too concerned with
	Hard to please	PERSONAL STANDARD		Easy-going
	Cool, aloof, withdrawn	PERSONALITY		Warm, accessible, sociable
	Very; get things done, work fast	PRODUCTIVE		Hard to complete tasks, slow
	Loner, self — conscious, feel awkward at large gatherings, socially inhibited	SOCIAL BEHAVIOR		Socially extroverted; love company, ritual, overt expressions of good form; amiable, easy going
	Tend to be antisocial, tend to try to get away quickly from social engagements or prefer not to go at all	SOCIALITY		Very sociable, people person, hate to be alone, love friendships and social interaction
	Excitable, fiery, hyper	TEMPERAMENT		Cool, calm, collected
	Angry, uptight, nervous, irritable, anxious, high-strung	TENDENCIES		Depressed, laid-back, lethargic, apathetic, easy going
	Quick	THOUGHT PROCESSES		Slow
	Workaholic, often take work home	WORK		Family oriented
		Psych Section Totals		
		Physical Section Totals		
		Diet Section Totals		
		GRAND TOTALS		

Final Words

Have your friends and family members take the MT Challenge and compare your results. When you're convinced that you are as unique on a biochemical level as you are in your fingerprints, the next step is to analyze your Metabolic Type® using the questionnaire outlined in the book, **The Metabolic Typing Diet: Customize Your Diet to Your Own Unique Body Chemistry** by Bill Wolcott or finding a Certified Metabolic Typing® advisor who will be able to do a more accurate computerised test.

A Metabolic Typing® advisors are now available in 40 countries. You can find a Certified Metabolic Typing® Advisors on the health excel website found in the resource section of the book (page 319) to read about their qualifications and available services.

I have been using Metabolic Typing® with my patients for many years now. You do not need to see an advisor in person. Metabolic Typing® evaluations and consulting can be done via e-mail and telephone.

The purpose of eating correctly for your Metabolic Type® is to balance body chemistry and maximize metabolic efficiency by properly addressing metabolic individuality. It is my belief that the presence of any degenerative disease (85% - 90% of diseases afflicting our population including scoliosis) is due to the failure to do just that. Thus, one way or the other, all degenerative disease has its origin in malnutrition.

The idea of malnutrition takes on an entirely different light when viewed through the perspective of Metabolic Typing®. We know that someone can eat the best organic foods and take the finest supplements that money can buy, yet still develop or fail to reverse degenerative disease. Time and again, we have seen that this can be due to the failure to meet one's genetically-based requirements for nutritional, biochemical balance.

CHAPTER 5

Ancient Bodies, Modern Diet

"Life in all its fullness is Mother Nature obeyed"

— *Weston A. Price, D.D.S.*

The foods that we eat in this day and age often do not bear even a passing resemblance to the foods that our ancestors ate. Today's modern foods, which include fast foods and processed foods, are not the kinds of foods our bodies are programmed to eat and digest. As a result, our bodies react to these unnatural foods by mounting an inflammatory response, which ultimately leads to the modern diseases we face today.

The cure to what ails us is to gradually alter our diet back to a closer approximation of what our bodies are genetically programmed to handle. This may sound difficult to achieve, but can actually be done quite easily.

In order to understand how we should eat in order to accomplish this, it is helpful to examine common diet patterns of the past, and how this shaped our genes over the course of many years.

In the early 1930's, a Cleveland dentist, Weston A. Price, (1870-1948) began to conduct a series of unique investigations to discover the root cause of disease and degeneration. Many refer to him as the "Albert Einstein of Nutrition." For over ten years, he traveled to isolated parts of the globe to study the health of populations untouched by western civilization. Among other things, he discovered that dental caries and deformed, crooked teeth are the result of nutritional deficiencies, caused by our modern-day, fast-food diets and are not the result of any virus, bacteria or inherited genetic defects.

Dr. Price's search for answers during the 1930's led him to launch a six-year expedition on five continents to study primitive societies in their natural habitat. The groups Price studied included isolated villages in Switzerland, Gaelic communities in the Outer Hebrides, indigenous peoples of North and South America, Melanesian and Polynesian South Sea Islanders, African tribes, Australian Aborigines and New Zealand Maori. This was a pivotal time, as there were still isolated tribes uninfluenced by civilization.

Indeed, when Dr. Price analyzed the foods consumed by these ancient tribes, he found that, in comparison to our modern day diet that is so influenced by the Western "fast-food" culture, these people used whole grains and natural (unprocessed) foods that provided almost four times the water-soluble vitamins, minerals and at least ten times the fat-soluble vitamins than those derived from modern diets. Dr. Price also discovered that these fat-soluble vitamins, vitamins A and D, were vital to health because they act as catalysts to mineral absorption and protein utilization. Lastly, Dr. Price was able to isolate a fat-soluble nutrient in their diets, which he named Activator X.

It was found that Activator X is present in fish livers, shellfish, and organ meats and butter from cows eating rapidly growing green grass in the spring and fall. All primitive groups had a source of Activator X, now thought to be vitamin K, in their diets.

He photographed these people and found that their strong body structures, ease of reproduction, emotional stability and freedom from various degenerative ills (heart ailments, diabetes and cancers to name just a few) are in sharp contrast to what Dr. Price referred to as "white man's diet" subsisting on the "displacing foods of modern commerce," that come saturated with heavy amounts of refined sugar, white flour, pasteurized milk, low-fat foods, vegetable oils and convenience items filled with artificial colors, flavors, preservatives and other additives.

Dr. Price's studies also discovered that the phenomenon of "borrowing," which is when the body is deficient in minerals and steals what it needs from the skeleton, which causes the skeleton to shrink over a certain period of time. Some people were reported to lose as much as 10 inches in height. This borrowing only occurred to those exposed to modern-day foods and not the aboriginal peoples he studied. Any wonder why people on a modern day diet tend to have weaker bones and are more prone to conditions like osteoporosis and scoliosis.

He also found that borrowing tended to occur more in females, particularly younger girls in the developmental stage of puberty and growth spurt. Because girls in modern societies are constantly bombarded with the image of beauty as being ultra thin, they often deprive their bodies of the nutrients they need to properly grow. The forming bones will borrow from bones that are already formed, particularly the spine. This leads to softened bones and a curvature of the spine, which explains why scoliosis affects more girls than boys.

The result of this disturbance of growth can often result in the lengthening of the body — meaning, modern-day dieters who aren't getting the proper nutrition are literally "skin and bone" as compared to those raised on a traditional diet because their skeletons are narrower due to borrowing. Again, this links scoliosis to diet as this body type is commonly seen among people who suffer from this condition.

The discoveries and conclusions of Dr. Price are presented in his classic volume, *Nutrition and Physical Degeneration*. The book contains striking photographs of handsome, healthy primitive people and illustrates in an unforgettable way the physical degeneration that occurs when human groups abandon nourishing traditional diets in favor of modern convenience foods. See these two set of photographs for evidence. No marks for guessing who is a child from a primitive race and who belongs to the modern, "civilized" world:

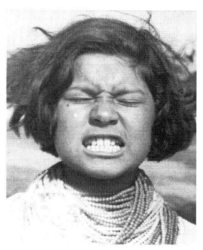 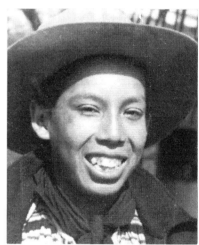

Copyright © Price-Pottenger Nutrition Foundation®. www.ppnf.org

Figure 7a: Saloman girl raised on nutrient-rich native foods

Figure 8a: Samoan girl was raised on a modernized diet.

Price's astonishing photographs — some 18,000 of them, supported his findings that societies living off primitive diets developed well-formed and strong structures such as teeth and facial features, while people living off a modern diet had developmental disorders such as increasingly deformed dental arches, crooked teeth, and cavities.

The Samoan girl in Figure 7a was born to parents who ate nutrient-rich native foods. The Samoan girl in Figure 8b was born to parents who had abandoned their traditional diet and adopted a more modernized diet. She has crowded dental arches and altered facial structure due to the effects of "borrowing" and will be more susceptible to dental decay and chronic illness.

In the words of Dr. Price: "We neither saw nor heard of a case (of arthritis) in the isolated (primitive) groups. However, at the point of contact with the foods from modern civilization many cases were found, including ten bedridden cripples in a series of about twenty Indian homes. Some other afflictions made their appearance there, particularly tuberculosis, which is taking a very severe toll on the children who have been born at the centre."[46]

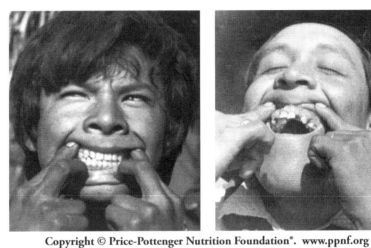
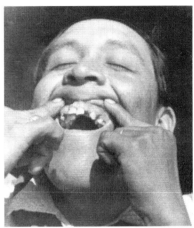

Figure 7b: Boy raised traditional native diet.

Figure 8b: Boy raised on a processed modernized diet.

In general, Dr. Price found that healthy isolated peoples, whose diets contained adequate nutrients from animal protein and fat, not only enjoyed excellent health but also had a cheerful, positive attitude to life. He noted that most prison and asylum inmates have facial deformities indicative of prenatal nutritional deficiencies.

The pioneering research of Dr. Price provides beyond a doubt the dangers of a modern diet. The primitive people he studied did not suffer from obesity, heart disease, arthritis, or scoliosis at the rate we do. Thanks in large part to their primitive diets, these people enjoyed levels of health that have been virtually lost to modern civilization.

The table on the next page explains the differences in traditional vs. modern diets that Dr. Price found in his research:

Traditional vs. Modern Diets

Traditional Diets Maximized Nutrients	Modern Diets Minimize Nutrients
Foods from fertile soil	Foods from depleted soil
Organ meats preferred over muscle meats	Muscle meats preferred, few organ meats
Natural animal fats	Processed vegetable oils
Animals on pasture	Animals in confinement
Dairy products raw and/or fermented	Dairy products pasteurized or ultra pasteurized
Grains and legumes soaked and/or fermented	Grains refined, and/or extruded
Soy foods given long fermentation, consumed in small amounts	Soy foods industrially processed, consumed in large amounts
Bone broths	MSG, artificial flavorings
Unrefined sweeteners	Refined sweeteners
Lacto-fermented vegetables	Processed, pasteurized pickles
Lacto-fermented beverages	Modern soft drinks
Unrefined salt	Refined salt
Natural vitamins occurring in foods	Synthetic vitamins taken alone or added to foods
Traditional cooking	Microwave, Irradiation
Traditional seeds, open pollination	Hybrid seeds, GMO seeds

Table 2: Courtesy of The Weston A. Price Foundation.

Processed Foods: Energy Dense But Nutritionally Poor

It will come as no surprise that many Americans have forsaken healthy and nutritious home-cooked meals in favor of high-calorie but nutrient-poor foods, including sodas and unhealthy snacks, according to studies of American eating habits over the past few decades.

What were once occasional indulgences has now become part of the regular mealtime fare of many Americans. Researchers have found a significant increase in meals composed of french fries, pizza, fried chicken, and burgers.

Over the past two decades, meal patterns have shifted from most meals being eaten at home to many meals eaten as fast or convenient meals from one of the numerous fast food outlets that have wildly proliferated.

Obesity and diabetes has reached alarming proportions, which can be attributed to two major causes: an increase in the amount of calories consumed in all age groups, combined with less physical activity. These two factors have proven to be a lethal combination.

Research from the U.S. Department of Agriculture, by Dr. Alanna Moshegh, studied changes in the popularity of favorite (and not-so-favorite) foods. She noted the following:

- A large increase in the consumption of unhealthy foods, such as burgers, pizza and chocolate
- Daily consumption of soda by children increased from 31% in 1970 to 46% twenty years later
- A replacement of healthy diet items such as low-fat milk, fruits and vegetables by nutrient-poor foods

The last three decades have brought changes to our lifestyle, an increase in the availability of fast-food restaurants, and an increase in the availability of processed "convenience" foods in supermarkets, leading to an increase in unhealthy eating habits that is becoming epidemic in proportions. Consider the following information regarding processed foods, which goes a long way towards explaining our seemingly insatiable appetite for processed foods and the results that can be expected:

Processed Foods are Addictive

Processed foods are foods that have been modified from their natural form, or their components have been concentrated. Changing or modifying these foods alters the way they are digested and used in your body. Dopamine is a neurotransmitter in your brain which, when stimulated by highly concentrated or processed foods, causes a pleasurable sensation. Therefore, eating these types of foods makes you feel good and gives you the allusion that they taste better, resulting in craving and addiction to these foods.

Processed Foods are More Likely to Cause Obesity

Certain additives in processed foods have been linked to weight gain and obesity (i.e. high fructose corn syrup, sugar).

Processed Foods Can Cause Imbalances in the Digestive System

Beneficial bacteria cannot thrive when they are constantly bombarded by foods that are difficult to digest, leading to digestive problems, illness, food cravings and disease.

Processed Foods Have Been Linked to Depression, Memory Loss, and Mood Disturbances

Fats and oils used in processed foods are stripped of their nutritive value, and do not contain the essential fatty acids needed for your heart and brain to function optimally.

Processed Foods Often Have Misleading Labels

Ingredients on processed food labels are often hidden or written in misleading terms. An example of this is when a label states the product is "sugar free," but contains sweeteners like agave, which is similar to high fructose corn syrup. Even savvy consumers can be fooled by these labels into a false sense of security.

Processed Foods Have Been Linked to Cancer

Processed meats, such as hot dogs and deli meats have been linked to cancers of the pancreas, colon, and stomach.

Processed Foods Have Been Linked to Infertility

A diet deficient in vitamins and minerals may be partially responsible for many cases of infertility. Infertility in the United States is on the rise. Many processed foods are stripped of the nutrients they originally contained.

Processed Foods are Manufactured for Long Shelf-Life

This means that chemicals and additives are added to processed foods to prevent them from spoiling on the grocer's shelf. These chemicals and preservatives can be harmful to your health.

The Most Important Nutritional Considerations for Growing Children

Teenagers are notorious for their poor eating habits, yet it is at this point in their lives that they most require adequate intakes of nutrients important to their growth, such as iron, vitamin D and calcium. Puberty, with its accompanying growth spurts, puts this population at risk for nutritional deficiency, especially in today's modern society, where healthy, nutritional food has been replaced with convenient processed and "junk" foods. The typical fare of today's adolescents is a drastic change from the food consumed by the adolescents that Dr. Price and other researchers studied.

Iron

Iron-deficiency anemia is common among adolescents for several reasons. Boys undergo a rapid accumulation of LBM (lean body mass) for each kilogram of weight that they gain. When they have finished growing, their LBM will be approximately double that of girls. For girls, weight gain and the onset of menses means that their iron needs become much greater than before puberty.

Increased muscle mass and blood volume during the growth spurt increases the need for iron to build up haemoglobin, which increases the oxygen-carrying capacity of the blood, as well as the protein myoglobin in muscle.

For these reasons, adolescents should be screened for iron deficiency. Foods that are high in iron, and should therefore be encouraged, include meats, dark green vegetables, beans and fish. The iron that is obtained from animal food sources (haeme iron) is much better absorbed, but the intake of vitamin C and animal proteins (i.e. meat and fish) can assist in the absorption of iron from non-animal sources, such as dark green vegetables. Teens that are vegetarian are at higher risk of iron deficiency which further risks scoliosis progression.

Calcium

Consider the following:

- Most of the gain in skeletal weight occurs during the adolescent growth spurt
- The skeleton contains at least 99% of the body stores of calcium
- Approximately 45% of the adult skeletal mass is formed in adolescence (although growth continues well past adolescence and into the third decade)
- The body cannot make calcium, so the growth of the skeleton is solely dependent on intake of calcium

When adolescents are growing rapidly, they only obtain calcium on an average of 200-300 mg per day. Because calcium is only partially absorbed (around 30%), it is important that the teen's diet contain enough calcium to build strong bones and avoid osteoporosis in later years. The recommended calcium intake can be achieved by adequate intake of dairy products, such as milk, cheese, and yogurt.

Vitamin D and phosphorus are also important in helping to build strong bones and is discussed in detail in chapter 11. As well, weight-bearing exercise stimulates the building and retention of bone mass. Regular exercise for 30 to 60 minutes per day, several days a week should be encouraged. Promoting healthy eating and exercise habits early in life will help entrench these health-promoting behaviors for a lifetime of healthy living.

Food Habits: Why Are Regular Eating Patterns And Snacks Important?

The habits of a lifetime are laid down in childhood and adolescence. This is why it is so important to teach and encourage good nutritional habits during this period.

Teenagers often develop poor eating habits, often skipping meals, especially breakfast. Studies have shown that children who eat a balanced, nutritional breakfast often perform better in school and are able to concentrate better than their peers who do not eat breakfast. Teens are also vulnerable to peer pressure to diet and become unhealthily slim, especially females.

In childhood, snacks are often offered periodically during the day, as children lack the capacity to eat large meals and thus become hungry between meals. The same is true for rapidly growing teens. Teens should be encouraged, both at home and at school, to choose healthy snacks.

Energy Needs of a Growing Child

Human beings are usually fairly adept at meeting their energy needs by moderating appetite, which is unconscious, and intake, which is under conscious control. Most teens are able to accomplish this balance, meeting their nutritional needs. However, teens are often vulnerable to a host of outside influences, which can negatively impact their appetite and eating patterns.

Teens are susceptible to stress, and although adults may feel that teen stress is relatively unimportant, it is very real to the teen experiencing it. They are especially sensitive to matters of physical appearance. Teens who have a negative body image may respond to emotional stress by under eating (dieting or starvation, which can lead to anorexia nervosa and other eating disorders) or overeating, leading to obesity. Obesity is a growing concern, and often persists into adulthood.

Recognition of destructive eating patterns is important, and teens who are very underweight or overweight should receive appropriate help from parents, their physician, or others knowledgeable in the field. Ignoring the problem may make it worse, and may lead to greater health problems in adulthood.

National surveys continue to demonstrate that the lack of Recommended Daily Amounts (RDA) of nutrients in our diets and increased intake of sugar-rich food is the leading cause of degenerative diseases. Research shows that these lifestyle diseases are almost absent in aboriginal societies. These diseases include coronary heart diseases, high blood pressure, degenerated disc, osteoarthritis, appendicitis, gallstone, diabetes, obesity, strokes, hemorrhoids, dental caries, all cancers and even scoliosis.

In fact, Dr. Price use to send modernized Eskimos and Indians attacked with tuberculosis, a fatal condition and untreatable with modern medicine, back to primitive conditions and to a primitive diet and found that a great majority recovered!

When Dr. Price studied the native diets, he noticed some similarities in the foods that were keeping them so healthy. Among them:

- The foods were natural, unprocessed, and organic (and contained no sugar except for the occasional bit of honey or maple syrup).
- The people ate foods that grew in their native environment. In other words, they ate locally grown, seasonal foods.
- Many of the cultures ate unpasteurized dairy products, and all of them ate fermented foods such as *natto, kimchi* or *kefir*.
- The people ate a significant portion of their food raw.
- All of the cultures ate animal products, including animal fat and, often, full-fat butter and organ meats.
- The native diets also had more omega-3 fat than modern diets and FAR less omega-6 fats. A diet that is lacking in omega-3 fats, and heavy on omega-6 fats from vegetable oils (which are consumed so heavily today) is a recipe for disaster.

Drug, Herbicide and Pesticide Exposure

In addition, drug, pesticide and herbicide exposure has been found to have a significant link to scoliosis in studies of animals. This leads to the suspicion that such an exposure may also be a leading cause of scoliosis in human beings; a suspicion that of course needs validation through scientific research.

So far, animal studies on scoliosis, drugs, herbicides and pesticides have led to the conclusion that:

- Kepone, a pesticide, is found to cause scoliosis in fish
- Pesticide exposure can caused spinal curvature in tadpoles
- Diquat, an aquatic herbicide, can cause scoliosis and other defects in duck embryos
- Large doses of ibutilide fumarate, an antiarrhythmic drug, can cause scoliosis in rat populations.

So how does one avoid all these dangers?

The decision to purchase organic food over commercially grown food is a personal one, and as you walk through the supermarket, you will note that many of them are now adding organic sections. Evidence now shows that chemicals that we are frequently exposed to in everyday life may increase health risks. This is especially important for children who are developing organs and a spine which must last them a lifetime. Due to their smaller bodies, faster metabolisms and less varied diets, infants and children are more vulnerable to health and developmental damage. By reducing toxic exposure, organic products can help us raise healthy, strong children.

What's Wrong with Politically Correct Nutrition

For starters, "politically correct" nutrition is not based on sound scientific evidence. On the contrary, it makes the following sweeping premises:

Myth: "Avoid saturated fats."

Saturated fats play many important roles in the body. They provide integrity to the cell wall, promote the body's use of essential fatty acids, enhance the immune system, protect the liver and contribute to strong bones. The lungs and the kidneys cannot work without saturated fat. Saturated fats do not cause heart disease. In fact, saturated fats are the preferred food for the heart. Because your body needs saturated fats, it makes them out of carbohydrates and excess protein when there are not enough in the diet.

Myth: "Limit cholesterol."

Dietary cholesterol contributes to the strength of the intestinal wall and helps babies and children develop a healthy brain and nervous system. Foods that contain cholesterol also provide many other important nutrients. Only oxidized cholesterol, found in most powdered milk, powdered eggs and hard boiled eggs, contributes to heart disease.

Myth: "Avoid red meat."

Red meat is a rich source of nutrients that protect the heart and nervous system; these include vitamins B12 and B6, zinc, phosphorus, carnitine and coenzyme-Q10.

Myth: "Cut back on eggs."

Eggs are nature's perfect food, providing excellent protein, the gamut of vitamins and important fatty acids that contribute to the health of the brain and nervous system. Americans had less heart disease when they ate more eggs. Egg substitutes cause rapid death in test animals.

Myth: "Eat lean meat and drink low-fat milk."

Lean meat and low-fat milk lack fat-soluble vitamins needed to assimilate the protein and minerals in meat and milk. Consumption of low-fat foods can lead to depletion of vitamin A and D reserves.

Myth: "Eat 6-11 servings of grains per day."

Most grain products are made from white flour, which is devoid of nutrients. Additives in white flour can cause vitamin deficiencies. Whole grain products on the other hand, can cause mineral deficiencies and intestinal problems unless properly prepared.

Myth: "Restrict salt"

Salt is crucial to digestion and assimilation. Salt is also necessary for the development and functioning of the nervous system.

Myth: "Limit fat consumption to 30 percent of calories."

Thirty percent of calories as fat is too low for most people, leading to low blood sugar and fatigue. Traditional diets contained 30 percent to 80 percent of calories as healthy fats, mostly of animal origin.

The bottom line is that not all fats are bad and some are essential for health. Depending upon your Metabolic Type®, you can figure out exactly how much fat is good for you and in what proportion you must balance it out with proteins and carbohydrates.

Eating the Diet of our Ancestors

When comparing the diets that were consumed by people in centuries past, it becomes obvious that the foods we consume now are very different from the foods that our ancestors ate. Our diet has changed to the extent that our bodies can barely recognize the foods that we eat, which is the major reason why we are susceptible to so many degenerative diseases these days.

Consider diabetes, the epidemic of our lifetime. Ancient diets contained very little sugar and refined starches, while our modern diet is overloaded with them. Our bodies respond to these alien chemicals and respond abnormally, by causing inflammation, obesity, and diabetes (which is really a by-product of obesity for most people).

Many of today's chronic diseases can be related to our consumption of foods foreign to our genes. Therefore, it makes sense that we should attempt to alter our diet until it more clearly resembles the diet that we are genetically pre-programmed to consume and can utilize wholly. This as discussed earlier in the book is the premise of Metabolic Typing® and an important step in stopping a scoliosis from progressing.

Personal Stories: Athlete Living with Scoliosis

"I had always had lower backache since I can remember. It was an ache that would come on after doing anything physical like house cleaning, sports, etc. And in rare occasions, it would ache even after doing none of those things. About October in 2007, I noticed that after physical activity not only my lower but also the middle of my back would ache. Then by January 2008, the ache I would get after physical activity had worsened. It got quite painful. From then on my back got worse. I kept being active, but it got hard to do. The middle of my back had started to give me huge discomfort when sitting down to study, watch TV, even to eat dinner. Then it got to the point where I was taking pain killers so that I could get to sleep at night. My back was hurting constantly. Come mid February, I decided that the pain was not going to go away by itself, that I must have something wrong, so I went and made an appointment with Dr Kevin. He sent me away to have X-rays. The next appointment, Dr Kevin showed me the X-rays and my spine was clearly crooked. I'm a young, fit, healthy, active individual and I very rarely get injuries so I kind of considered myself invincible in that aspect, so to see the state that my spine was in was a big reality check for me. I tried really hard to look after myself physically so I felt really disappointed that I had let this happen to myself and I wished I had done something about the pain earlier, because maybe then it would not have gotten so bad.

"During my 3 months of courses to relieve the pain, Dr Kevin had me take a questionnaire to see what Metabolic Type® I am. I am a fast oxidising protein type. He introduced me to a new diet that consisted of more protein and fat than what I normally eat. I was really dubious about it, fearful of the fat in the diet. But I gave it a go. For the first 2-3 weeks, I felt a bit sluggish and moody. The only good thing at that stage was that I did not feel hungry between meals anymore and found that I was snacking less. Then after about 4 weeks on the new diet, I started to really feel the benefits. My energy levels went up, I now sleep all night without waking up, I no longer have cravings for chocolate or cheesecake, I feel great and I have lost 3kgs without even trying to lose it."

Things I have learnt:

- Chiropractors are NOT scary and it does NOT hurt
- Back pain is NOT normal
- Some fats are NOT bad
- Some things it doesn't pay to be tough about. I should have addressed this problem a lot earlier

— *Isla W. (24 years old)*

Part 2

A Nutritional Program for Health and Scoliosis

CHAPTER 6

How is Nutrition Related to Scoliosis?

"One must eat to live and not live to eat."

— *Moliere*

Here I would like to make a very significant comment. If the band aid (signifying a quick-fix solution) for tooth decay is brushing and flossing your teeth daily, then band-aids for scoliosis is bracing.

Filling tooth cavities or opting for root canal treatment has the same implication as surgery for scoliosis, and nowhere is this more clearly illustrated than in Dr. Price's research. Dr. Price found and documented in his classic book *Nutrition and Physical Degeneration* that native tribes living on their traditional food nearly always had perfect teeth, and were almost 100 percent free of tooth decay. They were also almost entirely free of chronic diseases of the heart, lungs, kidneys, liver, joints, and skin. This is without the benefit of having toothbrushes, floss, toothpaste, or root canals and fillings, which is a remarkable feat for those days, and would be a miracle today!

However, when these tribal people were gradually introduced to sugar and white flour, guess what happened? Dr. Price tried it and their health, and their perfect teeth, rapidly deteriorated!

So while brushing and flossing — modern dentistry's mantra for healthy teeth — are important, they cannot be considered nearly as important a factor for healthy teeth as the food that you eat.

The real issue is diet. The natives that Dr. Price tracked down and studied weren't free of cavities, inflamed gums, and degenerative diseases because they had better tooth brushes! They just ate the food nature intended them to eat.

Ten Nutritional Principles to Better Health and Spine

Bracing and surgery, as mentioned earlier in this book, are helpful to an extent, but in the end, don't forget that they are merely band-aid options. For true and lasting health, you must really start at the basics and that means cleaning up your diet from the word go. The later chapters will explain these guiding principles in more details.

Guideline 1: Eat according to your ancestors or what your body has evolved to eat, your Metabolic Type®.

Guideline 2: Eat a variety of fresh, whole foods that will spoil, but eat them before they do.

Guideline 3: Eat a nutrient-dense diet to make every bite count. Avoid all processed foods which tend to be loaded with sugar, water, fat, flour, starch, artificial colorings and flavors.

Guideline 4: Eat a varied selection fresh vegetables and fruits, preferably organic, in salads or soups, or lightly steamed.

Guideline 5: Drink spring or filtered water as your main source of fluid. Limit sodas and processed fruit juices due to high sugar content.

Guideline 6: Eat traditionally fermented foods for a natural source of good bacteria (probiotics) and to optimise digestion.

Guideline 7: Prepare homemade meat stocks from bones or joints of chicken, beef, lamb or fish and use liberally in soups and sauces.

Guideline 8: Use whole grains and nuts that have been prepared by soaking, sprouting or sour leavening to begin to neutralize phytic acids and other anti-nutrients. Restrict or avoid refined carbohydrates and sugars, and limit your intake of all processed carbohydrates normally found in processed foods.

Guideline 9: Consume only healthy oils and fats which include extra-virgin olive oil, butter, flax seed oil, and fats from plant sources such as nuts, seeds, avocados, and coconuts. Animal fats from naturally raised livestock are also an excellent source of healthy fat.

Guideline 10: Minimize your consumption of highly refined vegetable cooking oils. Avoid all foods with partially hydrogenated vegetable oils and trans fats.

Research on Nutrition and Scoliosis

Believe it or not, scoliosis has been induced in a variety of animals through nutritional deficits and imbalances. As discussed before, many of the nutritional imbalances linked to scoliosis in animals, such as deficits of manganese, vitamins B6, and copper, have been found to have some potential to cause osteoporosis in human beings as well.

Past research shows that there are strong links between scoliosis and osteoporosis. This begs the question: Could nutritional deficiencies and diet also play a role in causing scoliosis in humans?

The answer is: It *seems* quite likely.

Here are some of the studies on nutritional imbalances and anomalies known to cause scoliosis in animal and human subjects:

- In chickens susceptible to scoliosis, the severity and incidence of scoliosis was decreased by giving the birds increased dietary copper. Later, in a clinical study on humans, teenage girls with scoliosis were found to have high levels of copper deposited in their hair. This led the authors of this study to conclude that copper may play a role in idiopathic scoliosis[47]

- Likewise, in another study on scoliosis in susceptible chickens, vitamin B-6, manganese or copper deficiencies caused an increase in the expression of scoliosis in the majority of the birds[48]

- Rainbow trout fed a diet deficient in ascorbic acid developed scoliosis[49]

- Channel catfish fed diets deficient in vitamin C developed skeletal malformations[50]

- Rats fed a diet deficient in vitamin E developed kyphoscoliosis[51]

- Salmon fed a diet deficient in vitamin C developed scoliosis[52]

- Trout fed diets containing excess leucine (an amino acid) developed scoliosis[53]

- In a study of humans with scoliosis, calcium was higher in idiopathic scoliosis muscles than in other forms of scoliosis or in normal control muscles. The authors suggested that a calcium-related neuromuscular defect could be an important factor in the genesis of idiopathic scoliosis

- Researchers in Hong Kong found that, "Inadequate calcium intake and weight-bearing physical activity were significantly associated with low bone mass in AIS (adolescent idiopathic scoliosis) girls during the peripubertal period. The importance of preventing generalized osteopenia in the control of AIS progression during the peripubertal period warrants further study"[54]

- Other research has focused on the importance of a number of nutrients such as, vitamin C, vitamin K, carnitine, CoQ10, glucosamine, magnesium and silica in the development of scoliosis in humans[55]

Dr. Paul Harrington, world-renowned orthopedic surgeon, suggests that a nutritional deficit and its associated hormonal influences during a young girl's vulnerable growing years may initiate the scoliotic process. Harrington states that, "during growth a balanced intake of proteins and vitamin C is essential to the support of normal collagen."

Patients with idiopathic scoliosis typically have manganese deficiencies, which along with reduced hyaluronic acid levels can lead to the development of elongated torsos.

Marginal deficiencies in manganese, zinc, copper, and pyridoxine have been shown to affect the expression as well as severity of idiopathic scoliosis. The highest incidence of idiopathic scoliosis occurs in the period of rapid growth that correlates with increased needs for manganese, zinc, copper, and pyridoxine. Manganese is essential to normal proteoglycan metabolism. Zinc tissue deficiencies result in defective collagen formation.

Small wonder that a recent study from researchers in Washington, D. C. found that nutrition should logically be considered as a possible factor in human scoliosis, based in part on a review of all of these studies in which nutrition appears to be playing a significant role in the disorder. At the end of the study the authors concluded that, "There is evidence that poor nutrition may play a role in the etiology of idiopathic scoliosis. This possibility should be examined further in humans."[56]

Research has proved beyond a doubt that scoliosis can result from various nutritional imbalances. Why is it that researchers have not come up with a "magic bullet" to cure scoliosis? The best they can do is manufacture various supplements in a feeble attempt to make up for the deficiencies present in many people's diets.

The primitive people that Dr. Price studied had no need of supplements because their diet supplied all that their bodies needed to prevent scoliosis from developing, and also to ward off many other diseases that plague our modern society. Their diets contained an ample supply of nutrients beneficial to their growth and development, and their consumption of foods that were cultured promoted the growth of natural and beneficial bacteria in their digestive tract, thus preventing many of the problems that modern people suffer from.

Your Health is Like a Tree

The missing piece of the puzzle in all of this research is that scoliosis is more than simply consuming enough nutritionally dense foods correct for your genetic type. It also entails proper digestion of whatever it is that you are consuming, so as not to cause any nutritional deficiency, such as the one referred to in detail by Dr. Price. A healthy gut flora provides 85 percent of our protection against disease. These two things - good food and good digestive health- go hand in hand.

Let me begin to explain that by giving you an analogy using the tree. Imagine your spine as being the trunk and your digestive system as being the root system. We all know that for a tree to grow strong and healthy it needs the right nutrients found in the soil, sufficient sunlight, clean water and air.

A growing person also needs the proper nutrients from food, sufficient sunlight, and other factors so that their spine will grow strong and healthy. What most forget is that even if the tree has all the right nutrients and factors for it to be healthy, if the roots are damaged then its ability to grow normally will be hampered. Therefore, if your ability to digest and assimilate food is compromised, your spine bends and health is compromised. It isn't just what you eat but also what you digest that determines your health.

I often explain to my patients that there are two stages of healing: eating correctly for your Metabolic Type® and digesting correctly. What I've observed with my scoliosis patients is that they generally tend to be extremely thin, yet have the ability to eat and eat without putting on weight. These people have to be built up from the inside out as their bodies are not efficient in digesting and absorbing what they consume. The progress that I observe with them is remarkable, to say the least, even after a few months of dietary adjustment that corrects any digestive problems.

I use the word 'adjustment" because what I propose is not something very radical. I propose practical, everyday solutions, except that they are tuned in to the individual's unique needs for optimal spinal growth. The right kind of foods ultimately also improves their mood patterns and promotes a general feeling of well-being.

Good Digestion is a Prerequisite for Spinal Health

Alternate medical practitioners have always known it, scientists however, have only just begun to find the evidence to prove that bone health is also related to gut health.

A paper published in the journal *Cell* by Dr. Gerard Karsenty, M.D., Ph.D., chairman of the Department of Genetics and Development at the Columbia University College of Physicians and Surgeons, reports that nearly 95% of serotonin, a neurotransmitter that can controls bone formation, is produced in the gut and only about 5% in the brain. Until now, the skeleton was thought to control bone growth, and serotonin was primarily known as a neurotransmitter acting in the brain.[57]

However, the relationship between bone formation and serotonin — the "happy" chemical that's responsible for alleviating depression through its activity in the brain — is an inverse one: the less serotonin in the gut; the denser and stronger our bone structures. The opposite is also possible: the higher the level of serotonin, the more brittle the bones become. In extreme cases, the result can be bone disorders such as osteoporosis and scoliosis. Could poor digestion and lack of good bacteria be the cause for less serotonin to be absorbed into the body? It seems quite likely.

"This proof-of-principle paper shows, to our amazement, that bone formation is regulated to a significant extent by the gut!" stated Dr. Karsenty'.

While science is slowly catching up with the natural medicine philosophy that there is a definite link between nutrition, gut health and skeletal development.

Remember, Not All Bacteria Are Bad Bacteria

Bottom line is, even if the proper food for your Metabolic Type® or genetic requirement is eaten and the proper supplements are taken, it is quite another for that food and those nutrients to be absorbed into your body. In other words, just because a food goes down your esophagus, it does not mean that the nutrients will make it to your cells. First, digestion must prepare the food to enable it to penetrate the wall of your intestines. But if the food does not encounter the proper acid, enzymes and good bacteria, it will not digest and thereby will not absorb properly, potentially causing malnourishment, as well as making your body fertile ground for the development of degenerative diseases.

In fact, research has now demonstrated that the type of bacteria that you carry in your digestive system also affects how efficiently (or inefficiently) you assimilate your food. Even more impressive is evidence that proves the nutritional cause of many diseases is related to an imbalance of bacteria in your gut, a problem easily rectified by eating correctly for your Metabolic Type®, taking a high quality probiotic and adding fermented foods to your diet.

Dr. Price's research was consistent with the research of Dr. Francis Marion Pottenger, a medical doctor and author of *Pottenger's Cats*. In his classical experiments in cat feeding, more than 900 cats were studied over 10 years, Dr. Pottenger demonstrated that consumption of pasteurized milk or cooked meats resulted in a rapid onset of disease and bodily malformation. Dr. Pottenger found that only diets containing raw milk and raw meat produced optimal health: good bone structure and density, wide palates with plenty of space for teeth, shiny fur, no parasites or disease, reproductive ease and gentleness.

His clinical observations suggested that a similar process also occurs in humans. The implications for western civilization, obsessed as it is with refined, highly sweetened convenience foods and low-fat items is profound. Based on his findings, Dr. Pottenger stated, "Nutrition becomes one of the most important elements in preventative medicine."

In other words, regardless of which disease process is being studied, the link between poor nutrition and disease, including scoliosis, clearly exists in studies and my own clinical observations of hundreds of patients.

Personal Story: Healing from the inside out.

"I first learnt my spine has a sideway curve eight years ago when I went for a full body massage. The masseuse traced the curvature with her finger. I dismissed it as an abnormality I was probably born with and thought no more of it as I had no pains nor aches anywhere. However, in the past few years, I suffered from tense shoulders and low energy.

"A few months ago, I began to wonder whether my symptoms were all connected to my scoliosis. Dr. Kevin Lau performed a visual assessment and sent me for X-rays which confirmed I had right thoracic "C" shaped scoliosis of 36 degrees from the neck to mid back. Dr. Kevin's scoliosis correction program taught me how to do certain exercises to stretch and strengthen muscles of my spine. Treatment also involved exercises and decompression therapy at each session.

"Besides the exercises and spinal manipulations, Dr. Kevin emphasises the importance of providing our muscles, joints and bones with the necessary nutrients to get better. He also encourages us to rid our bodies of unwanted organisms (bad bacteria) and to make our own probiotics to improve our digestive systems. With more probiotics in our digestive systems, our cells will be able to absorb more of the nutrients we're sending their way and be healthier.

"Over a period of six months, X-rays of the earliest patients have been very encouraging. All the patients treated by Dr. Kevin Lau have had their curvatures reduced. There was a 15 year old girl who improved from 45 degrees to 28 degrees and a 70 year old from 16 degrees to 4 degrees. I know how much my spine improved as it showed a 10 degree correction from 43 deg to 33 degrees and I certainly feel much more relaxed. Dr. Kevin Lau has a passion for getting his patients well."

— *June T. (34 years old)*

CHAPTER 7

Introduction to Fermented Foods

"All diseases begin in the gut."

— *Hippocrates (460-370 BC)*

Did you know that...

- All traditional diets consume healthy lacto-fermented foods and beverages every day to help to keep digestive systems balanced
- The fermentation process increases the nutritional value of the foods we eat and makes it easier to digest
- Fermented foods recolonize your digestive system with beneficial bacteria and help the scoliosis sufferer assimilate their food
- The friendly bacteria in fermented foods are significantly less expensive than probiotics and can be found in greater numbers than are typically present in any pill or supplement
- Cultured vegetables are wonderful for controlling sugar cravings
- Fermented products are a great source of amino acids, vitamins, and minerals
- Last but not least, fermented products can kill helicobacter pylori (the ulcer causing bacteria) and other pathogenic bacteria

Though the term "fermented" sounds vaguely distasteful, the results of this ancient preparation and preservation technique that involves the breakdown of carbohydrates and proteins by microorganisms such as bacteria, yeasts and molds — are actually delicious. These foods have been around for thousands of years, but we have never needed them more than we do today.

The Dutch seaman used to carry sauerkraut on long voyages to prevent scurvy. For centuries, the Chinese have consumed cultured cabbage during the long winter months to ensure a source of green vegetables throughout the winter. Kefir, a cultured dairy drink from Tibet (or the Caucasus mountains) and Natto, from Japan (made of fermented soya beans), are regularly consumed by some of the longest-living societies in the world. Coincidence? I don't think so.

These fermented foods are so nutritious that some of these are now considered to be "functional foods" which promote the growth of friendly intestinal bacteria, aiding digestion and supporting immune function, producing B vitamins (including Vitamin B12), vitamin K, digestive enzymes and lactic acid, and other immune chemicals that ward off harmful bacteria and cancer cells from your bodies.

Getting Proactive With Probiotics

Would you believe that recent research by a bunch of Finnish scientists indicates that the types of bacteria present in a baby's gut may determine their risk of being overweight or obese later in life?

After analyzing fecal samples from 49 infants, 25 of whom were overweight or obese by the age of 7, they found that babies with high numbers of bifidobacteria and low numbers of Staphylococcus aureus appeared to be protected from excess weight gain.

In addition, they discovered that breast-fed babies are at a lower risk of turning obese as bifidobacteria flourish in the guts of breast-fed babies.

Source: American Journal of Clinical Nutrition
March 2008, Vol. 87, No. 3, 534-538

Traditional Fermentation Cannot Be Found on Supermarket Shelves

The key phrase you must watch for on food labeling if you want to achieve the amazing health benefits of fermented foods is "traditionally lacto-fermented", as not all of these tasty condiments from the supermarket are created equal.

Fermentation is an inconsistent process — more an art than a science — so commercial food processing techniques are used for more consistent yields. Technically, anything that is "brined" in salt stock is fermented, but that's where the similarity ends, as each type of fermented food has specific, unique requirements and production methods.

Refrigeration, high-heat pasteurization and vinegar's acidic pH all slow or halt the health promoting enzymatic processes.

For example, if you leave a jar of pickles fermenting at room temperature on the kitchen counter, the gas produced by the live bacteria would probably blow off the lid and cause the jar to explode. Can you imagine the problem this would cause on a supermarket shelf? This is why, all "shelf-stable" pickles also have to be pasteurized and lack the beneficial bacteria in them.

You may be surprised to learn that our primitive and traditional diets always carried a high content of food enzymes and beneficial bacteria from lacto-fermented vegetables, fruits, beverages, dairy products, meats and condiments. When soaked, sprouted and fermented, seeds, grains, and nuts neutralize naturally occurring anti-nutrients such as enzyme inhibitors, tannins and phytic acid.

People with scoliosis are usually deficient in various vitamins and minerals because their body's use of these nutrients depends on adequate levels of friendly bacteria in the intestinal tract. When traditionally fermented foods are included in the diet, your body will soon be populated with sufficient amounts of these needed bacteria.

Four years ago, the World Health Organization reported that the Japanese, who consume large amounts of fermented soy foods like *natto* and *miso* along with green tea, ginger and ocean herbs, enjoy the longest lifespan in the world!

In the same study, modernised cultures like America didn't even make it to the top 20. Could it be because of what they are eating and their sedentary lifestyle habits?

A typical modern Western diet, as we all know, is mainly comprised of fast, convenient, processed and genetically altered foods. Is it any wonder that problems like heart disease, obesity, autism, and scoliosis are steadily on the rise there?

The bottom line is fermented foods are essential for health as they help to normalize cholesterol, strengthen your digestion and immune systems, and proactively help fight off all manner of diseases including scoliosis.

Fermentation for the Modern Ages

Unfortunately, the art of making fermented produce has been lost, due to the time and effort involved. That is why I use (and highly recommend to my patients) a top-quality starter culture which supplies the beneficial bacteria to the food you are fermenting. Traditionally, these starter cultures were not necessary, as these bacteria were handed down from one generation to the next, such as in the form of kefir "grains." These days they are difficult to obtain and the art of fermentation is almost extinct.

A "culture starter" product, however, is a very easy way to make cultured vegetables, yogurts and even sour cream (i.e. traditionally fermented foods, not the unhealthy "imposter" versions displayed on almost all supermarket shelves.). Adding a "starter culture" ensures that your food begins fermenting with a hardy strain of beneficial bacteria. The culture starter contains a very robust probiotic bacteria that preserves key nutrients, vitamins, and antioxidants; while eliminating toxic components from food and destroying a number of potential pathogens in the gut.

I recommend to my patients that they experiment and choose a few fermented foods that they like and gradually add them into their daily diet.

Some of the fermented super-foods that we are going to discuss in this section include:

- Kefir
- Sauerkraut
- Kimchi and
- Natto

What is Kefir?

Kefir, which literally translated means "feel good" in Turkish, is an ancient cultured, enzyme-rich food filled with friendly micro-organisms that help balance your "inner ecosystem" to maintain optimal health and strengthen immunity.

The world of lacto-fermentation is indeed a fascinating one. Virtually every culture has some kind of fermented food or beverage that could be significant sources of amino acids, vitamins and minerals. They produce substances that inhibit harmful bacteria such as salmonella. They can eradicate H. Pylori, the bacteria responsible for the majority of gastric ulcers. In this series, I will talk about a few of the ferments with which I have become very familiar over the last several years. When all is said and done, fermentation is not only cheaper and better than popping a probiotics pill, but is also a lot healthier for you.

Kefir is a dairy ferment. For vegetarians it's considered to be the mother culture of all dairy ferments. I regard kefir grains to be Probiotic-Jewels and their culture-product kefir a Probiotic-Gem. This view is shared by Jordan Rubin in *The Maker's Diet*, who relied on kefir and other dietary habits to heal from Crohns, a severe intestinal disease.

Throughout history, kefir was readily consumed in the Caucasus Mountains. The Caucasus peoples enjoyed longevity of over 100 years. There is a legend that kefir grains were a gift of the prophet Mohammed, and they fiercely guarded their grains for fear they would lose their strength if given away and the secret of making kefir got out. Even Marco Polo mentioned it. Yet the magical properties of kefir were forgotten for centuries until news spread of its successful use in the treatment of tuberculosis, intestinal and stomach diseases. The first studies on kefir were published in Russia at the end of the 19th century.[58]

Traditionally, kefir is prepared by fermenting milk with kefir grains. The word 'grains,' however, is a misnomer, as they look like little pieces of cauliflower and have absolutely no relationship to cereal grains. They are composed of a firm gel-like mass of proteins, fats and polysaccharides and reproduce in a dairy medium. However, they are difficult to find as they are passed from one friend to another.

Also the organisms may vary between different grains. Indeed the culture starter is what differentiates between "very good", "good" and "average" value kefir.

Commercial powdered starters are also available and these contain 10-15 organisms, while the bottled kefir you buy in the store contains a maximum of 10 strains (along with a lot of sugar you don't want). Most bottled kefir contains only bacteria as many states do not allow the selling of beverages with live yeasts, so if you want kefir for its probiotic value, it only makes sense to culture your own. It is very simple to do, taking about five minutes a day. It is also quite simple to prepare cheese from kefir.

Kefir has a creamy consistency with a slightly tangy (sour) taste depending on how long it's been fermented. Mine often gets as thick as yogurt. Many, if not most people, drink kefir after culturing for 24 hours then straining. However, by doing this, they are missing out on many of the benefits of kefir. For example, by ripening kefir another 24 hours, the content of folic acid is increased 116%.

Apart from kefir's obvious probiotic value, it possesses other healing properties. Research in Japan found that rats with tumors that were fed kefir grains, had reductions in tumor size. Kefir is also proving to have anti-inflammatory properties. In 2003, the anti-inflammatory effect of kefir was investigated and correlated scientifically by Prof. Jose M. Schneedorf et al. Other research shows regularly eating the kefir can lower blood pressure, cure constipation, and control blood glucose.

Kefir's tart and refreshing flavor is similar to a drinking-style yogurt, and it contains beneficial yeast as well as the friendly 'probiotic' bacteria found in yogurt. When used regularly, the naturally occurring bacteria and yeast in kefir combine symbiotically to help balance your intestinal flora and boost your immunity. Among its many beneficial powers, kefir:

- Provides supplemental nourishment for pregnant and nursing women*
- Contributes to a healthy immune system
- Promotes a relaxing effect on the nervous system and benefits many who seek a restful night's sleep
- Helps support your normal intestinal tract function, promotes bowel movements and a healthy digestive system — and is beneficial after the use of antibiotics to restore balance to the digestive tract

- Curbs unhealthy food cravings by making your body more well-nourished and balanced

While kefir will work with all milk, even powdered milk, it does like a little fat. Many experts recommend organic fresh milk (cow or goat) from grass-fed animals. If you can't get organic milk, try and find milk that is free of hormones or antibiotics. Above all, avoid ultra pasteurization and powdered milk as it is the most damaging to the structure of the milk proteins, making it difficult to digest. Again, kefir grains or starter cultures will do their magic with any milk.

If you are lactose intolerant, the initial 24-hour fermentation will remove about 50% of the lactose, which is the food for the organisms. Ripening the kefir after straining for an additional 24 hours at room temperature or for several days in the refrigerator, will remove almost all the lactose.

A small study published in the May, 2003, *Journal of the American Dietetic Association* showed that drinking kefir eliminated - or, at least, dramatically reduced - symptoms of lactose intolerance in 15 adult participants. Researchers at Ohio State University tested plain kefir, raspberry-flavored kefir, plain yogurt, raspberry-flavored yogurt and two-percent milk in this group after a 12-hour fast. The participants recorded any symptoms of lactose intolerance after consuming each food. They reported few or no symptoms after ingesting both types of kefir and both types of yogurt.

Kefir vs. Yogurt

While both kefir and yogurt are cultured milk products, they contain different types of beneficial bacteria. Yogurt contains "transient" beneficial bacteria that keeps your digestive system clean and provides food for the friendly bacteria that are already present. Kefir actually helps to colonize your intestinal tract — a feat that yogurt cannot match.

Additionally, kefir contains several major strains of friendly bacteria not commonly found in yogurt: Lactobacillus Caucasus, Leuconostoc, Acetobacter species, and Streptococcus species. It also contains beneficial yeasts, such as Saccharomyces kefir and Torula kefir, which help balance the intestinal flora, including promotion of beneficial yeast in the body by penetrating the mucosal lining. They form a virtual SWAT team that housecleans and helps strengthen the intestines.

Kefir's active yeast and bacteria may provide more nutritive value than yogurt by helping digest the foods that you eat and by keeping the colon environment clean and healthy. The curd size of kefir is smaller than yogurt, so it's also easier to digest, making it an ideal food for babies, the elderly, and anyone with digestive health concerns.

Did you Know?

A healthy adult on an average carries 1.5 - 2 kg of bacteria in his gut? Fortunately, all this bacteria is not bad. Some is indeed good and beneficial for our health. So good in fact, that were our gut to be completely sterilized, we might even die!

Kefir: A Nutritional Powerhouse for Bone

The exceptional nutritional content of kefir offers a wealth of healthy benefits to people with any type of condition and especially to scoliosis patients. More than just beneficial bacteria, kefir contains minerals and essential amino acids that help your body access its natural healing powers and maintenance functions. The complete proteins in kefir are partially digested and therefore more easily utilized by the body.

Tryptophan, which converts to serotonin, the feel good chemical in the brains abundant in kefir, is well-known for its relaxing effect on the nervous system and more recently in its importance in bone formation. It also offers loads of phosphorus, calcium and magnesium - all of which are essential in normal growth and development of the musculoskeletal system. In any case, all scoliosis sufferers will benefit greatly from incorporating kefir into their regular dietary habits.

Making Your Own Kefir

Ingredients

- 50 grams (1¾ oz) of kefir grains or kefir starter culture
- 500 ml (1 pint) fresh milk

Preparation:

- Remove kefir grains from previous batch of starter, using a sieve or colander.
- Shake kefir grains to remove excess kefir. Rinsing is not necessary (but optionally, rinse in fresh milk).
- Place kefir grains in glass jar or jug with fresh milk. Generally, keep a ratio of kefir grains to milk of about 1:10.
- Set aside to ferment at room temperature for up to 24 hours.

Note: Non-milk kefir can be made from sugary water, fruit juice, coconut juice, rice milk, or soy milk. However, the kefir grains will stop growing in these liquids, so it is best to only use excess kefir grains or powdered kefir starter for this.

Personal Story: A Dad Finds Kefir Beneficial for Scoliosis

"Since my two daughters began drinking kefir milk, we have seen tremendous improvement in their overall health. They both used to be very sickly. My youngest suffered from allergies and asthma and my oldest suffered from scoliosis.

"I am absolutely certain that since they started drinking kefir, they haven't been sick except for an occasional cold that only lasts a couple of days instead of the normal bout that would last for weeks with trips to the hospital and all kinds of antibiotics and steroids.

"After just a month of drinking kefir milk, we noticed changes in our daughters immediately. My youngest daughter's asthma attacks were becoming less frequent. Before, she used to be at the doctors almost every two weeks for her asthma. To date, she has not had an asthma attack in more than 20 months now!

"When I think back now, after reading about the long-term negative effects that antibiotics and steroids can have from Dr. Kevin Lau's blog, I can't help but wonder if they had something to do with my older daughter's scoliosis. After taking so many different kinds of drugs, she would get better for about three weeks at the most, and then she would get sick again and the cycle would just repeat itself. It's such a relief to see my daughters enjoying a healthy life now thanks to kefir milk. It's true that prevention is definitely the best medicine and a good diet is a much cheaper and healthier alternative."

— *Edgar D. (46 years old)*

Cultured Vegetables

I now present another "super" food that can contribute immensely to healing and building your digestive system.

Raw cultured vegetables have been around for thousands of years, although we have never needed them as much as we do today. Rich in lactobacilli, enzymes and loaded with vitamins, they are an ideal food that can and should be consumed with every meal.

Benefits of Cultured Vegetables

Raw cultured vegetables help re-establish your inner ecosystem. The friendly bacteria in raw cultured vegetables are a less-expensive alternative to probiotics.

- They improve digestion
- They increase longevity

You might think of the friendly bacteria in raw cultured vegetables as little enzyme powerhouses. By eating the vegetables, you will maintain your own enzyme reserve and use it to eliminate toxins, rejuvenate your cells, and strengthen your immune system which all adds up to a longer, healthier life. Additionally:

- They control cravings
- They are ideal for pregnant and nursing women
- Raw cultured vegetables are alkaline and very cleansing

Meanwhile, cultured vegetables also help restore balance if your body is in a toxic, acidic condition. Because they do trigger cleansing, you may have an increase in intestinal gas initially as the vegetables stir up waste and toxins in the intestinal tract. Soon, however, you will notice an improvement in your stools.

Believe it or not, recently scientists have also discovered a cure for the deadly bird flu (avian influenza) in the fermented vegetables.

Professor Kang Sa-ouk of Seoul National University said in an interview with the Associated Press, that South Korea had begun to sell an extract of *kimchi* to treat the flu outbreak. This product is widely used throughout the world, and it is wonderful that a natural extract might be the key to treating this deadly disease, but if people were to go back to their "roots" and begin consuming traditionally fermented vegetables, there may not be a need for an expensive extract.

Two Cultured Vegetables Recipes

1. Traditional Sauerkraut

Ingredients:

- One fresh medium-sized cabbage, red or green
- Non-chlorinated water
- Vegetable "starter culture"

Preparation:

- Shred the cabbage either by hand or with a food processor.
- Place the shredded cabbage in a large bowl.
- Pound the cabbage.
- Mix 1 packet of vegetable culture starter to the filtered water.
- Place pounded cabbage and juices in a medium sized glass jar. Press down firmly on the cabbage while pouring cultured water to the jar until cabbage is fully submerged. The mixture should be at least one inch from the top of the jar.
- Cover the jar and let it sit for 3 to 7 days at room temperature.
- After it is fermented, store it in the refrigerator.

Once in the fridge, it can last 2-3 months due to the preservation method used. Vegetables such as carrots, cauliflower, wakami, chili and ginger can be added to make it more interesting.

2. Kimchi (Korean Sauerkraut)

Ingredients:

- 1 head of cabbage, cored and shredded
- 1 bunch of green onions, chopped
- 1 cup of carrots, grated
- 1/2 cup of daikon radish, grated (optional)
- 1 tablespoon ginger, freshly grated
- 3 cloves of garlic, peeled, crushed and minced
- 1/2 teaspoon of dried chili flakes
- 1 tablespoon of ocean sea salt, i.e. "Celtic Sea Salt or Himalayan"
- 1 packet of vegetable culture starter

Preparation:

- Place vegetables, ginger, red chili flakes, ocean sea salt and water made with the starter culture in a bowl and pound it with a wooden mallet to release the juices.
- Put it all in wide-mouth jar with a tight-fitting lid.
- Press down firmly with a mallet until the juices rise to the top of the mixture. The juice should completely cover the vegetables, and the top of the juices and mixture should be at least 1 inch below the top of the jar, to allow room for expansion.
- Screw the cover on tightly and keep it at room temperature (68 to 77 degrees Fahrenheit) for 3 days (72 hours).
- After 3 days, it should be kept in the refrigerator or some other cold place.

What is Natto?

Often compared to cheese because of its pungent aroma, natto is composed of steamed soybeans that are fermented until they acquire their "nutty" flavour. Natto has a slippery-sticky paste on its surface, and once stirred, the slippery paste increases in volume, forming spider web-like threads. Since it's an "acquired taste," fans of blue cheese will probably love natto.

Natto has been a traditional Japanese food for more than 1,000 years. According to Japanese folklore, the famous warrior Yoshiie Minamoto was responsible for introducing natto to north western Japan. Ancient Samurai consumed natto on a daily basis and even fed it to their horses to increase their speed and strength. During the Edo Period (1603 - 1867), natto was given to pregnant women to insure a healthy newborn.

Natto is produced by a fermentation process, by adding Bacillus natto, a beneficial bacterium, to boiled soybeans. For centuries, it was easily made at home; soybeans were packed in straw (which contained a natural bacillus) then buried for a week in the ground. Today, natto is made by injecting the bacteria. The Bacillus natto acts on the soybeans, producing the nattokinase enzyme. Other soy foods contain enzymes, but only the natto preparation contains the specific nattokinase enzyme.

When compared to ordinary soybeans, the natto produces more calories, fibre, calcium, potassium and B2. Natto has slightly less protein than beef, but contains more fibre, iron and nearly double the calcium and vitamin E.

Natto is Food for Your Bones

Natto is high in calcium, B vitamins and soy isoflavones, but the real benefits of natto, flow directly from it being a rich source of vitamin K. Vitamin K is absolutely essential to build strong bones and also helps promote heart health. For several years, compelling evidence has shown that most people don't get enough vitamin K to protect their health through the foods they eat.

Green leafy vegetables supply almost half of the vitamin K requirement for the majority of Americans. Most foods considered rich in vitamin K have shown to have less vitamin K than previously thought. Despite this vital information, the majority of multi-vitamins don't contain any vitamin K at all and those that do don't contain enough.

Recent research supporting vitamin K's usefulness in bone and heart health is now becoming too abundant to overlook. Still, very few health-conscious consumers understand the importance of supplementing vitamin K.

While other nutrients are important for maintaining bone health, there is increasing evidence indicating the significant role of vitamin K in bone metabolism and healthy bone growth. New studies have also emerged that link Vitamin K to joint and cartilage health as well. Insufficient vitamin K in the body has been associated with osteoarthritis and can result in poor bone and cartilage mineralization. The study found that people with high levels of vitamin K were less likely to develop bone spurs, joint-space narrowing, and osteoarthritis. This research suggests that eating a diet rich in Vitamin K can help slow or even stop the progression of osteoarthritis altogether.[59]

Vitamin K has been linked to cells that generate or "lay down" bone and produce a specific protein that acts as a kind of glue helping to incorporate calcium into the bones. Vitamin K2 is necessary in order to produce this protein.

Research shows that vitamin K regulates calcium in the bones and arteries, promoting heart health and bone health at the same time. Vitamin K seems to do the impossible, accommodating the needs of both bones and arteries.

Here is a simple explanation: Proteins that don't get enough vitamin K can't hold on to the calcium, either. Without a functioning protein to control it, calcium drifts out of your bones, into your arteries and other soft tissues. Vitamin K gently redirects the "lost" calcium back to the bone "bank".

One ground-breaking study observed the change in circulating vitamin K and Gla osteocalcin (used for bone mineralization) concentrations in normal individuals with the intake of natto. Volunteers were divided into three groups. One group received regular natto, while the other two groups were given natto fortified with two varying concentrations of vitamin K.

Among the experimental group, it was discovered that bone nutrients were significantly higher at seven, ten and fourteen days after the start of the fortified natto. Similar beneficial effects were not observed in the case of volunteers taking regular natto, although vitamin K levels were found to be significantly raised.

These findings suggest that although regular natto is also effective reinforced natto, which contains more MK-7 than regular natto, would be just the kind of food that patients with scoliosis would need for their bone health. We will discuss vitamin K supplementation in greater detail later in the book.

Natto is more difficult and time-consuming to make at home. However, for those too busy, commercial natto is available in some Asian groceries in the Japanese frozen food isle. Usually it is sold in sets of three or four 50-gram packages. I recommend taking 1 -2 packets per day for scoliosis sufferers.

I am sharing the recipe below. But be warned that for the uninitiated it smells bad, and is an acquired taste. Those wanting to get the benefits of vitamin K without the hassle can take the supplement form discussed in chapter 11.

Homemade Natto

Ingredients:

- Two cups of dried soybeans
- Water
- One package commercial natto or a packet of bacillus natto starter culture

Preparation:

- Soak two cups of dried soybeans overnight in ten cups of water.
- Put the soybeans in a stainless steel basket (or colander) and cover them with a piece of cloth slightly larger than the basket.
- Pressure cook with 3 cups of water for 15 minutes.
- In the meantime, have a package of commercial natto ready.
- Open the lid of the pressure cooker, peel back the cloth cover to one end of the basket, and using the tablespoon, and quickly mix in about two spoonfuls of natto starter with the beans. Replace the cloth cover.
- Close the pressure cooker lid with its air relief hole uncovered.
- Place an electric heating pad over the cooker and allow it to ferment for 24 to 48 hours, depending on the temperature of the heating pad.

CHAPTER 8

Essential Carbohydrates

"I give you bitter pills in sugar coating.
The pills are harmless: the poison is in the sugar."

— *Stanislaw Jerzy Lec*

In the search of creating the perfect diet, carbohydrates are often listed as a culprit to good healthy eating. Carbohydrates are popularly known as the energy source of food eaten by humans and animals. The "energy" comes from a rise in the metabolism caused by eating carbohydrates, which consist of starches, sugars, celluloses and gums. Carbohydrates come in two forms: simple and complex. Simple carbohydrates are found in foods such as candy, fruit, and baked foods, while complex ones are found in starch foods like vegetables, beans, whole grains, and nuts.

The world's culture has become very dependent on foods such as potatoes, grains, rice and others, which has helped to feed and grow a large population, just look at China, but the problem is the amount of carbohydrates consumed by an individual. The problem with carbohydrates is that they turn to glucose, which feels good at the beginning as the metabolism is raised, but it also releases insulin, adrenaline, and cortisol, which are known to cause diseases such as heart disease, diabetes, cancer, strokes, blood clots, as well as diseases of other organs such as eyes, kidneys, blood vessels, and nerves. And now we are just learning of the detrimental effects it can have on spinal health and scoliosis.

Nutrition specialists, such as Dr. Loren Cordain, suggest that 2-3 grain servings per day per individual would be beneficial to most, less would be better. Carbohydrates are not essential for survival. It is more important to have the protein, fat, water and minerals in a body's system rather than carbohydrates.

History has shown that humans were not made to digest high carbohydrate foods, but rather high protein foods such as animals that would be hunted for and eaten. In the beginning of the agricultural era, there undeniably were many benefits in helping supply food to many nations, helping permanent communities to survive and the establishment of civilization. The fossil record indicates that early farmers, compared to their hunter-gatherer predecessors had a characteristic reduction in stature, an increase in infant mortality, a reduction in life span, an increased incidence of infectious diseases, an increase in iron deficiency anemia, an increased incidence of softening of the bone, osteoporosis and other bone mineral disorders and an increase in the number of dental caries and enamel defects.

Dr. Joseph Brasco, a medical doctor and researcher states:

> "In a review of 51 references examining human populations from around the earth and from differing chronologies, as they transitioned from hunter-gathers to farmers, one investigator concluded that there was an overall decline in both the quality and quantity of life.

> There is now substantial empirical and clinical evidence to indicate that many of these deleterious changes are directly related to the predominately cereal-based diets of these early farmers. Since 99.99% of our genes were formed before the development of agriculture, from a biological perspective, we are still hunter-gathers."

Early agriculture did not bring about increases in health, but rather the opposite. It has only been in the past 100 years or so with the advent of high tech, mechanized farming and animal husbandry that the trend has changed.

Dangers of Excess Carbohydrates

Centuries ago, people hunted and gathered their food. The foods that they had access to consisted of lean meats, seafood, and vegetables that were not subjected to the ravages of pesticides, as most of our vegetables are today. Their diet was a high protein, low carbohydrate and low saturated fats diet.

In order to find and gather foods, hunter-gatherers had to be in top physical condition. The amount of exercise they engaged in stimulated their bodies to increase the number of muscle cells, and the number of mitochondria (the "power plants" of the cells) within muscle cells. Hunter-gatherers were not subject to becoming obese, as people are today.

In modern times, we also forage for foods, but only so far as the nearest fast-food outlet or grocery store replete with packaged and processed foods. Our diets have become high in sugar and refined carbohydrates. We eat high quantities of saturated and trans fats, but consume little in the way of quality proteins, vitamins, and minerals. Our meals are generally calorie-dense but nutrient-poor.

When we consume large quantities of empty carbohydrate calories, the result is high glucose levels in our bodies. This, in turn, stimulates the secretion of insulin. Insulin is a hormone whose purpose is to move sugar into cells to supply energy for our body requirements. Insulin, however, has other roles besides providing sugar to our cells for energy, it also has implications for our genes and our cells beyond that of sugar metabolism. High insulin levels stimulate fat accumulation around the waist, stimulate our appetite, and increase the risk of heart disease, cancer and even scoliosis. Insulin increases levels of cortical, a stress hormone known to accelerate aging, and also increases the production of C - reactive protein, which also speeds up aging and promotes inflammation. A little- known fact is that insulin also controls the amount or calcium and magnesium gets stored in the body. If insulin levels are too high, though, the body loses calcium and magnesium—with urinary output. They just passes through without going to areas the body needs it, including the muscles and bones. Therefore keeping your insulin levels low is essential for good spinal health. Following the dietary recommendations in this chapter can help you to achieve a fasting insulin under 12 mcIU/ml of blood, which is considered ideal. Some scientists even advocate keeping your insulin levels as low as 8 mcIU/ml.

Sugar: Sweet Poison

Apart from corn, most people are addicted to sugar, and along with grain addiction, the over-consumption of added sugar is one of the major health problems facing all modern societies today. Sugars are simple carbohydrates processed by the body in the same manner as grains. That is, any excess sugars in the body are converted by insulin into fat — and just like grains, we're consuming an excessive amount of sugar.

I classify refined sugar as a poison because it has been depleted of its life forces, vitamins and minerals. What is left in the refining process is nothing but carbohydrates. The body cannot utilize this refined starch and carbohydrates unless the depleted proteins, vitamins and minerals are also present in combination. You would simply not be able to metabolize the carbohydrates in isolation. (Even if you could, there would be the side effects of an excess presence of these carbohydrates).

Incomplete carbohydrate metabolism begins to generate pyruvic acid, which starts accumulating in the brain, other parts of the central nervous system and your red blood cells, causing great havoc there. These toxic metabolites can interfere with your cell respiration. Cut off from oxygen, the cells gradually begin to die.

That's the reason doctors regard refined sugar as "lethal." It provides you nothing but "empty" or "naked" calories. It lacks the natural minerals which are present in the sugar beet or cane.

In addition, sugar drains and leaches your body of other useful vitamins and minerals that your body demands. These include important minerals such as sodium (derived from salt), potassium and magnesium (from vegetables), and calcium (from the bones).

Beware of Sugars and Grains

A recent Agence France-Presse report labels India and China as the diabetic capitals of the world, with the numbers of sufferers worldwide expected to grow more than 50 percent by 2025.

Paul Zimmet, a pioneering diabetes researcher and foundation director of the International Diabetes Institute in Melbourne, Australia told the AFP report[60] that the number of people with Type Two diabetes is expected to increase from 250 million last year to 380 million by 2025.

The most common cause of Type 2 diabetes is obesity caused by poor diet and a lack of exercise. The disease has become rampant in both developed and developing countries as a result of traditional diets being abandoned for processed and junk foods and people getting less exercise. In China, where more than 40 million people have Type 2 diabetes or its precursor, its prevention has become a national health priority.

If you made no other adjustments to your diet but eliminating or vastly reducing grains and sugars, it is likely your health would rapidly improve and within days you'd start losing weight. No matter what your health condition or Metabolic Type®, you are strongly advised to eliminate or restrict your grain and sugar intake, particularly processed grains and sugars. Eliminating grains is especially necessary for those who are Protein Types who tend to be genetically inclined to pre-agricultural foods. Carbohydrate and Mixed Types can get by with consuming a limited amount of whole grains as they are better genetically adapted to the grains, legumes, and especially flour products which were introduced due to modern agriculture. In all cases, any grains you do consume should be whole grains (95% of the grains consumed in the US are processed, which strips them of what limited nutritional value they do have).

It is primarily your body's response to the overindulgence of grain and sugars, not your intake of fat, which makes you overweight. Consuming sugar also leads to an accumulation of bad bacteria and fungus begins to proliferate in your digestive system, which can impair your white blood cell function, thereby decreasing your body's immune system and making you more vulnerable to diseases of all kind. Your body has a limited

Fats vs. Carbohydrates

Dietary fat, whether saturated or not, is not a cause of obesity, heart disease, or any other chronic disease of civilization. The problem is the carbohydrates in the diet, their effect on insulin secretion, and thus the hormonal regulation of the human body. The more easily digestible and refined the carbohydrates, the greater the effect on our health, weight, and well-being.

capacity to store carbohydrates, but it can easily convert those excess carbohydrates, via insulin, into body fat, which means the more excess carbohydrates you consume, the more body fat you will store.

Corn: The Forgotten Grain

Most people can easily name the common grains such as rice, wheat, oats, barley, and rye but forget that corn also belongs in that category, as they perceive corn to be a vegetable. Corn is a grain, and is relatively high in sugar, which is one of the main reasons it is America's number one crop. It consumes over 80 million acres of US land and sneaks its way into an endless array of food (and other) products. In its unprocessed or 'whole' state, corn offers negligible health benefits at best; sweet corn, for instance, contains vitamin C. You are best served by avoiding corn in its processed state.

Food with labels containing corn derivatives such as corn syrup, fructose, high fructose corn syrup, corn oil, corn meal, cornstarch, dextrose, monosodium glutamate, xanthan gum, and maltodextrin have no place in your grocery cart. Corn sweeteners are actually now the most widely produced of all sweeteners, accounting for 55% of sweeteners on the market. This is primarily high fructose corn syrup, which is the dominant ingredient in soft drinks, cookies, candies, and other popular grocery store items. Consumption of high-fructose corn syrup increased from zero in 1966 to a whopping 62.6 pounds per person in 2001, and is a key culprit in the diabetes and overweight epidemic.

Excess Carbohydrates Bad for Bones

Bone health is greatly dependent upon the controlled consumption of carbohydrates in the body. The body reacts greatly to the increase or decrease of carbohydrates in the system. Hypoglycemia episodes can be caused by the increased discharge of insulin in the blood stream through the extreme proportion of carbohydrates to protein. When carbohydrates are digested into the system at an increased level, while protein is decreased in consumption, the ratio creates an increased level of insulin into the body, because the blood level regulatory system in the body is fighting to keep blood levels normal. When the adrenal glands become involved in the process, they begin to produce cortisol and adrenalin. Excessive cortisol causes many unwanted responses in the body such as decreased cellular use of glucose, lessened protein synthesis, demineralization of the bones which can lead to osteoporosis, decreased lymphocyte numbers and functions, may cause more allergies, infections and degenerative diseases from lessened secretory antibody productions (SIgA), blood sugar will be increased, along with protein breakdown causing muscle wasting, and the skin regeneration and healing of the body will be affected.

Bone minerals are easily washed from our system by eating too many carbohydrates. This process can happen as the mineral makeup in the body is removed from the body extracting high-tensile strength collagen protein fibers from bones caused by high cortisol levels. This also weakens the connective tissues at the joints. Osteoporosis and degenerative disc disease are often found where the body has created too much cortisol through eating excessive carbohydrates and not enough protein. One inch can be lost in height in a year. Bones become more brittle and can break easily as well as hip fractures becoming more possible.

Women have been told for many years to increase their calcium intake to protect their bones by drinking more milk and eating more yogurt. This prescription to good bone health will not work because if carbohydrates are increased in the system from the lactose in milk and yogurt, along with the fruits and sugar in the yogurt, which encourages the loss of bone minerals rather than building onto it. The yogurt is normally store bought and high in sugar, but making your own ferments such as kefir or yogurt solves this.

If you really need sugar, stevia is a good substitute as it is the safest sweetener to use. It is a natural herb originating from South America that has been used for 1,500 years, and has been shown to be very safe. It is several hundred times sweeter than sugar, so you don't need much, but more importantly, it does not raise insulin or adversely affect your spinal development.

The only way to have a balanced healthy diet and prevent the loss of bone minerals is to minimise the amount of simple carbohydrates and eat complex carbohydrates appropriate for your Metabolic Type ®.

Healthy Carbohydrates to Eat

There is no food group that is denser with vitamins, minerals, antioxidants, and flavonoids than the vegetable group. This is particularly true for the vegetables that grow above the ground. Vegetables provide the good carbohydrates you need, and much more. Those who are Protein Types should ideally get most of their carbohydrates from vegetables, with virtually none from refined grains or sugar added foods. Those who are Carbohydrate Types, should ideally derive the bulk of their carbohydrates from vegetables but can also do well with about 15% of their carbohydrates derived from healthy, whole grains. Mixed Types, as the name implies, fall in the middle of these two.

The glycemic index is a measurement of how quickly food breaks down into glucose. Because more vegetables are high in fibre and low on the glycemic index, and are packed with nutritional value, vegetables are an ideal way to meet your daily carbohydrate requirements.

Guidelines to Choosing Vegetables

Carrots and corn are the two most frequently consumed vegetables; however, another study found that potato chips and French fries made up over one-third of children's diets. With vegetable intakes like this, it is easy to understand why so many kids are sick.

For health purposes, pretend that potatoes are not a vegetable but are instead grain. The reason for this is because they are high in simple carbohydrates and they act upon your body similar to grains and sugars, promoting weight gain and disease. French fries are double trouble, high in dangerous trans fats and you should avoid them like the plague.

Limit your consumption of other root vegetables, such as beets and carrots, as they are higher in carbohydrates than above-ground vegetables. If you do eat them, eat them raw as cooking increases their glycemic index.

While it is true that vegetables are a healthy part of any balanced diet, containing valuable nutrients, minerals and vitamins, some vegetables are better than others.

If you are trying to increase your consumption of vegetables, choose wisely. For example, iceberg lettuce has almost no nutritional value, being composed mainly of water. A far better option is romaine lettuce or spinach, which is high in iron.

If you choose to use organic vegetables, try to find the freshest organic vegetables available i.e. those grown locally. If you cannot find organic vegetables near you, fresh vegetables are always a better choice than canned or frozen vegetables. In addition, fresh vegetables should be washed to remove dangerous pesticides.

Fruit is Not as Healthy as Many Claim

Fruit is not the healthy food many claim. Fruit is mostly fructose sugar with some vitamins, minerals and other nutrients. Those vitamins and nutrients are easily obtained from meat and non-starchy vegetables without the fructose. The body processes fructose from fruit in the same way as it processes fructose from soft drinks. There is no difference. Fructose is fructose no matter what the source. Fructose causes insulin resistance as proven in scientific tests. Fructose is highly addictive and most people simply refuse to give up fruit no matter how sick they become. This is identical to lung cancer patients who continue to smoke cigarettes.

How Much Carbohydrate Should You Eat?

So how does someone know if they can tolerate more carbohydrates in the form of grains? How do they know which ones suit them best?

This is where Metabolic Typing® will come in. Finding out your Metabolic Type® will determine how much your body can process carbohydrates. Most people don't do very well when the total caloric intake of grains approaches 70% even carbohydrate type. For some of these people, it means lowering carbohydrate intake to below 40%, sometimes even as low as 20%. By moderating carbohydrate intake you can increase your fat burning as an optimal and efficient source of almost unlimited energy.

I suspect that for most people, a simple subjective test can be conducted in which they reduce the amount of grains in their diet and replace the grains with more vegetables and meats and seafood and a moderate amount of fruits based on your Metabolic Type®.

CHAPTER 9

Proteins the Bodies Building Blocks

"The best and most efficient pharmacy
is within your own system."

— *Robert C. Peale*

Despite what many fad diets out there have insisted upon, you need a certain amount of carbohydrates, protein and fat in your regular diet. None of these are as evil as some 'experts' have made them out to be. The key is to first, recognize and choose only the healthiest types of each of these and second, consume the right amount for your personal Metabolic Type®.

Proteins are the "building blocks" for the body which are required for nutrition, growth and repair, and affect a huge number of metabolic, enzyme and chemical processes that occur inside the body.

Protein actually consists of smaller units called amino acids, which link together in a variety of differing combinations to perform unique functions. Some amino acid chains are created by the body, but some - essential amino acids - must come from outside the body, from the food that we eat. Although all animal and plant cells contain some protein, the amount and the quality of the protein varies considerably.

Vegetables contain the majority of the micronutrients (vitamins, minerals, fiber and photochemicals) your body needs. However, there are essential macronutrients that vegetables cannot provide sufficient quantities of, including protein with all eight essential amino acids, found only in animal products and certain fats such as omega-3 with EHA and DPA fatty acids. Vegetables also contain a host of essential nutrients that are not found or replicated in any other type of food and certainly not in any pill or supplement.

If you do not have insulin challenges or are a carbohydrate type, then legumes in moderation can be a nutritious food source as they are rich in both fiber and minerals. Legumes are also high in vegetable protein, but you should be aware that their protein is incomplete, as it does not contain all eight of the essential amino acids your body needs. Animal protein such as fish, meat, eggs, and dairy is the only source of complete protein and therefore vegetarians should consume some animal protein like dairy, non-toxic fish, or eggs to prevent protein deficiency.

Everyone — irrespective of their Metabolic Type® — needs good protein. Carbohydrate Types a little, Mixed Types need more and Protein Types need considerably more. The best source of protein is meat. Does this mean vegetarians shouldn't be vegetarians? No, but if you are a vegetarian, be sure that you are a carbohydrate type and to include dairy, eggs and fish in your diet as only animal proteins provide all the essential amino acids and micronutrients your body requires to function at its highest level.

In terms of the red meats you can eat with confidence, grass-fed beef is an outstanding health value plus what most people agree is incredibly tasty.

Real Beef is Grass Fed

Until the mid-20th century, the vast majority of beef was pasture raised and fed a diet of native grasses. That's not the case today: the cattle industry quickly discovered that grain-fed animals bulked up quicker, allowing them to go to market at 14 or 15 months instead of four or five years. This accelerated market cycle translated to profits, and the worldwide cattle industry has never looked back.

But there's one big problem. Cows can't digest corn. Just as humans who eat an excess of grains and sugars can develop disease, the same happens to cows.

Cows, like other grazing animals, are ruminants. This means they have a rumen, or a 45-gallon-sized stomach that ferments grass, converting it into protein and fats. Ruminants are not physically equipped to digest grain. Switching a cow from grass to grain opens the floodgates to a host of serious maladies, including the presence of E. coli, which only a constant diet of antibiotics can begin to counter.

Raised on the cow's proper diet of grass, it is leaner than grain-fed beef. In fact, grain- fed beef can have an omega 6:3 ratio higher than 20:1.[62] This amount well exceeds the 4:1 ratio where health problems begin to show up because of the essential fat imbalance. Also, grain-fed beef can have over 50% of the total fat as the far less healthy saturated fat.

Grass-fed beef has an omega 6:3 ratio of 0.16 to 1. This is the ratio science suggests is ideal for our diet. This is about the same ratio that fish has. Grass-fed beef usually has less than 10% of its fat as saturated fat. If you are a pregnant or breastfeeding mom, the extra omega 3 from the grass fed beef will provide incredible nutritional benefits for your child.

In sum, it's now proven beyond doubt that, grass-fed beef, unlike grain-fed beef, is:

- A natural source of omega 3 fats
- High in CLA (conjugated linoleic acid)
- High in beta carotene
- Contains 400% higher amounts of vitamins A and E
- Virtually devoid of risk of bovine spongiform encephalopathy (mad cow disease)

In addition, grass-fed beef is also loaded with other natural minerals and vitamins. Lastly, it's a great source of CLA (conjugated linoleic acid), a fat that reduces the risk of cancer, obesity, diabetes, and a number of immune disorders.

Beware of organic grain-fed beef. Although it may be organic, the cattle are fed grains and grains are NOT what cattle are designed to eat.

Safe Fish to Eat

Fish is one of the healthiest meats you can eat as it is an exceptional protein source with high amounts of the omega 3 fats.

However, the majority of the fish that you buy at supermarkets and restaurants, most likely came from a fish farm. Not surprisingly, fish farming, a multimillion-dollar industry, has become one of the fastest-growing sections of the food production market.

What many people don't know is that farmed fish face many of the same health issues as factory-farmed animals. In order to be profitable, fish farms must raise large quantities of fish in confined areas, and the overcrowding leads to disease and injuries to the fish. The fish are given antibiotics and chemicals for the parasites like sea lice, skin and gill infections and other diseases that commonly affect them.

The fish are also given drugs and hormones, and sometimes are genetically modified, to accelerate growth and change reproductive behaviors. Farmed salmon are also given chemicals, canthaxanthin and astaxanthin, to turn their flesh pink in order to make them more marketable. Wild salmon eat a diet of shrimp and krill, which contain natural chemicals that make the salmon pink. Farm-raised salmon do not eat a natural diet, so their flesh would be gray if they were not given the additives.

If you do eat farmed fish try limiting it to only a few meals a month and try to choose from the following six safest fish: Wild Pacific Salmon, Snapper, Striped Bass, Sardines, Haddock and Pacific Flounder.

Eat Your Eggs

A section of people steer clear of eggs altogether. That is a dangerous trend in my opinion. What they may not know is that eggs do not cause an increase in cholesterol. Nor do they increase the risk of heart disease.

Eggs are considered one of nature's perfect foods, containing all known nutrients except vitamin C.

They are a good source of fat-soluble vitamin A and D that protect against free radicals and are important for the growth and development of a child. When possible, buy eggs from chickens that are allowed to roam free and eat their natural diet. There is a world of difference between the nutrient levels of eggs laid by free-range pastured hens vs. commercially farmed hens.

Ideally, when you are eating eggs, the yolks should be consumed raw as heat will damage many of the highly perishable nutrients in the yolk. Additionally, the yolk has cholesterol that can be oxidized with high temperatures, especially when it comes in contact with the iron present in the whites, and is cooked as in scrambled eggs.

Preparing the Perfect Protein

Foods that are high in protein, such as fish, chicken, lean meats and eggs are broken down during the process of digestion into amino acids. These amino acids are then transported to where they are needed in the body, where genes provide the blueprints for recombining these amino acids into specific substances your body needs in order to function properly.

Protein-rich foods, such as those mentioned, are also high in vitamins B6 and B12, are needed to manufacture and repair our cell's DNA.

Protein-rich foods from animal sources are your best bet because they are complete proteins, containing all eight essential amino acids. Protein from vegetable or other sources are likely to be incomplete sources, and may be high in things you don't want, such as carbohydrates. These sources of protein may not be your best bet if you are trying to maintain or lose weight.

Omega-3 fats, which most people are lacking in their diet, can be found in eggs, turkey, lean beef and pork, and chicken. Animals which have been grass-fed or that are free range will have higher levels of omega-3 fats and low levels of saturated fats, something you may want to keep in mind when choosing your protein.

In general, faster and lighter cooking methods, such as stir-frying, are preferable because they produce fewer Advanced Glycation End products (AGEs), which can be damaging to the body in excessive amounts. Similarly, cooking in a liquid, such as poaching fish in water, limits AGE production. Thus, steaming, poaching, and rapid pan-frying and stir-frying are superior to grilling and baking. However, baking food in a broth or coating food with olive oil before baking will reduce the formation of AGEs.

Personal Story: Learning to be Proactive with my Scoliosis

"I was eleven years old when I discovered I had scoliosis through a routine school exam. My curvature was 10-20 degrees and not deemed significant enough to require a brace or surgery. Doctors continued to monitor me every six months, with no noticeable deterioration. I was lucky that I never was forced to wear a brace. Once through puberty I was eventually discharged and told my spinal condition had stabilized. At this point I suffered no pain or discomfort.

"Years later when I started working, I started to suffered from backaches after sitting or standing for prolonged time. I sought treatment at a local hospital and was prescribed glucosamine. The doctor attributed the pain to pressure on the spine due to the curves, and I was advised not to do any impact sports like jogging and playing basketball. As these were my primary exercises, I suddenly felt like I couldn't exercise anymore. I simply stopped being active for fear of the pain.

"By this time my curvature had progressed to 39 degrees. My doctor took annual X-rays to monitor the deterioration. I was told if the curvature passed 45 degrees then surgery was the only option available. Plagued by backaches, I feared trying any exercises, even if they were prescribed. Two years later I tried various therapies for pain relief. Although they did help ease my pain level, they did nothing to correct my curvature. I noticed absolutely no relief from the glucosamine. I honestly felt that it was inevitable I would eventually need surgery. I felt helpless, and with little hope for any solution.

"I am so thankful that I met Dr. Kevin Lau before my spine deteriorated any more than it already had. He restored my hope with his exercises and diet information. As I completed his exercises my core muscles also gained a tremendous amount of strength which strengthened my spine. My right curvature decreased from 39 degrees to 30 degrees and my left curvature went from 28 degrees to 27 degrees. The back pain and stiffness significantly diminished which allowed my activity level to improve. I no longer lived in fear of movement which used to lead to horrible pain. I feel that I can finally be proactive about my scoliosis rather than just sit around and monitor the changes and wait for surgery.

"Dr. Lau restored my hope in my life, and I no longer see the need for surgery in my future."

— *Isabel C. (34 years old)*

CHAPTER 10

The Truth about Fats

"To eat is a necessity, but to eat intelligently is an art."

— La Rochefoucauld

To begin with, let's demolish a few myths associated with fats:

Myth #1: Heart disease is caused by consumption of cholesterol and saturated fat from animal products while a low-fat, low cholesterol diet is healthier for people.

Truth: During the period of rapid increase in heart disease (1920-1960), American consumption of animal fats declined, but consumption of hydrogenated and industrially processed vegetable fats increased dramatically *(USDA-HNIS)*.

The Framington Heart Study is often cited as proof of this myth where residents of Flamington, Massachusetts, who ate more saturated fats, cholesterol and calories had the lowest serum cholesterol levels.

Myth #2: Saturated fat clogs arteries.

Truth: Studies have shown that the fatty acids found in artery clogs are mostly unsaturated (74%), of which 41% are polyunsaturated *(Lancet 1994 344:1195),* and not the saturated fats of animals or plant such as coconut.

Myth #3: Animal fats cause cancer and heart disease.

Truth: Statistics say the opposite. The fear of butter and animal fat has lead to the drop in consumption in the last century, but the incidence of heart disease and cancer has skyrocketed.

Animal fats contain many nutrients that protect against cancer and heart disease; elevated rates of cancer and heart disease are associated with consumption of large amounts of vegetable oil *(Federation Proceedings July 1978 37:2215).*

Myth #4: Children benefit from a low-fat diet.

Truth: Children on low-fat diets suffer from growth problems, failure to thrive and learning disabilities *(Food Chemistry News 10/3/94).*

Myth #5: A low-fat diet will make you "feel better...and increase your joy of living."

Truth: Low-fat diets are associated with increased rates of depression, psychological problems, fatigue, violence and suicide *(Lancet 3/21/92 Vol 339).*

Myth #6: To avoid heart disease, we should use margarine instead of butter.

Truth: Margarine eaters have twice the rate of heart disease as butter eaters *(Nutrition Week 3/22/91 21:12).*

Myth #7: Asians do not consume enough essential fatty acids (EFAs).

Truth: Asians consume far too much of one kind of EFA (omega-6 EFAs found in most polyunsaturated vegetable oils), but not enough of another kind of EFA (omega-3 EFAs found in fish, fish oils, eggs from pasture-fed chickens, dark green vegetables and herbs, and oils from certain seeds such as flax and chia, nuts such as walnuts and in small amounts in all whole grains) *(American Journal of Clinical Nutrition 1991 54:438-63).*

Myth #8: The "cave man" or "hunter and gatherer" diet was low in fat.

Truth: Throughout the world, primitive peoples sought out and consumed fat from fish and shellfish, water fowl, sea mammals, land birds, insects, pigs, cattle, sheep, goats, game, eggs, nuts and milk products *(Abrams, Food & Evolution 1987).*

The fact of the matter is that some fats can actually help you stay thin, improve your metabolism, and improve your immune system regardless of your Metabolic Type®.

Bad Fats to Avoid

However, regardless of your Metabolic Type®, the following newfangled fats can cause cancer, heart disease, immune system dysfunction, sterility, learning disabilities, growth problems and osteoporosis:

- All hydrogenated and partially-hydrogenated oils
- Industrially processed liquid oils such as soy, corn, safflower, cottonseed and canola
- Fats and oils (especially vegetable oils) heated to very high temperatures in processing and frying.

Trans Fatty Acid

An unhealthy substance, also known as trans fat, made through the chemical process of hydrogenation of oils. Hydrogenation solidifies liquid oils and increases the shelf life and the flavor stability of oils and foods that contain them. Trans fat is found in vegetable shortenings and in some margarines, crackers, cookies, snack foods and other foods.

Trans fats are also found in abundance in "french fries." To make vegetable oils suitable for deep frying, the oils are subjected to hydrogenation, which creates trans fats. Research suggests that amounts of trans fats correlate with circulatory diseases such as atherosclerosis and coronary heart diseases and should be avoided.

Vegetable Oils

Myth: "Use more vegetable oils."

Truth: Polyunsaturates in more than small amounts contribute to cancer, heart disease, autoimmune diseases, learning disabilities, intestinal problems and premature aging. Large amounts of polyunsaturated fats are new to the human diet, due to the modern use of commercial liquid vegetable oils. Even olive oil, a monounsaturated fat considered to be healthy, can cause imbalances at the cellular level if consumed in large amounts.

The Truth about Saturated Fat

Saturated fats, such as butter, meat fats, coconut oil and palm oil, tend to be solid at room temperature. In conventional wisdom, these traditional fats are to blame for most of your modern diseases — heart disease, cancer, obesity, diabetes, malfunction of cell membranes and even nervous system disorders like multiple sclerosis.

However, many scientific studies indicate that it is processed liquid vegetable oil — which is laden with free radicals formed during processing — and artificially hardened vegetable oil — called trans fat — that are the culprits in these modern conditions, not natural saturated fats.

Humans need saturated fats because we are warm-blooded. Our bodies do not function at room temperature, but at a tropical temperature. Saturated fats provide the appropriate stiffness and structure to our cell membranes and tissues. When we consume a lot of liquid unsaturated oils, our cell membranes do not have structural integrity to function properly, they become too "floppy," and when we consume a lot of trans fat, which is not as soft as saturated fats at body temperature, our cell membranes become too "stiff."

Contrary to the accepted view, which is not scientifically based, saturated fats do not clog arteries or cause heart disease. In fact, the preferred food for the heart is saturated fat; and saturated fats lower a substance called Lp(a), which is a very accurate marker for proneness to heart disease.

Fats have been demonized in the United States, says Eric Dewailly, a professor of preventive medicine at Laval University in Quebec. The Inuit's diet is that more than 50 percent of the calories in Inuit native foods come from fats. Yet they don't die of heart attacks at nearly the same rates as other Canadians or Americans says Dewailly.

Much more important, the fats come from native wild animals, not farm raised. Farm animals, cooped up and stuffed with agricultural grains (carbohydrates) typically have lots of unhealthy fats which is not naturally seen in wild animals. Much of our processed food is also riddled with trans fats, such as the reengineered vegetable oils and shortenings cached in baked goods and snacks.

Saturated fats play many important roles in the body chemistry. They strengthen the immune system and are involved in inter-cellular communication, which means they protect us against cancer. They help the receptors on our cell membranes work properly, including receptors for insulin, thereby protecting us against diabetes. The lungs cannot function without saturated fats, which is why children given butter and full-fat milk have much lower rates of asthma than children given reduced-fat milk and margarine. Saturated fats are also involved in kidney function and hormone production.

Saturated fats are required for the nervous system to function properly, and over half the fat in the brain is saturated. Saturated fats also help suppress inflammation. Finally, saturated animal fats carry the vital fat-soluble vitamins A, D and K2, which we need in large amounts to be healthy.

Human beings have been consuming saturated fats from animal products, milk products and the tropical oils for thousands of years; it is the advent of modern processed vegetable oil that is associated with the epidemic of modern degenerative disease, not the consumption of saturated fats.

Healing With Coconuts

Coconuts are high in saturated fat that, contrary to popular belief, is a necessary fat for optimal nutrition. There are three different types of saturated fat, and coconuts contain the healthiest type, with medium-chain fatty acids that will actually help you lose weight while increasing health!

Since coconut oil contains a high proportion of saturated fats, some doctors may conclude that it's bad for your heart. However, research into coconut oil has discovered that it is indeed good for the heart.

A study in the 2004 edition of Clinical Biochemistry found that coconut oil, especially virgin coconut oil, lowered cholesterol, in particular LDL (bad) cholesterol, while raising HDL (good) cholesterol.

Likewise, an epidemiological study featured in *The American Journal of Clinical Nutrition* examined two indigenous populations whose food energy was 63% and 34% derived from coconuts and found no elevated risk of vascular disease.

The medium-chain fatty acids (MCFA) abundant in coconuts are digested more easily and utilized differently by the body than other fats. Whereas other fats are stored in the body's cells, the MCFA in coconut oil is sent directly to the liver where it is immediately converted into energy. So when you eat coconuts and coconut oil, your body uses it immediately to make energy rather than store it as body fat. Because this quick absorption puts less strain on the pancreas, liver and digestive system, the oil in coconuts 'heat up' your metabolic system which will burn more calories in a day — contributing to weight loss and more energy.

Fat-Soluble Vitamins for Growth

The crux of Dr. Price's research has to do with what he called the "fat-soluble activators," vitamins found in the fats and organ meats of grass-fed animals and in certain sea-foods, such as fish eggs, shellfish, oily fish and fish liver oil. The three fat-soluble activators are vitamin A, vitamin D and vitamin K2, the animal form of vitamin K. In traditional diets, levels of these key nutrients were about ten times higher than levels in diets based on the foods of modern commerce, containing sugar, white flour and vegetable oil. Dr. Price referred to these vitamins as activators because they serve as the catalysts for mineral absorption. Without them, minerals cannot be used by the body, no matter how plentiful they may be in the diet.

Modern research completely validates the findings of Dr. Price. We now know that vitamin A is vital for mineral and protein metabolism, the prevention of birth defects, the optimum development of infants and children, protection against infection, the production of stress and sex hormones, thyroid function, and healthy eyes, skin and bones. Vitamin A is depleted by stress, infection, fever, heavy exercise, exposure to pesticides and industrial chemicals, and excess protein consumption.

Modern research has also revealed the many roles played by vitamin D, which is needed for mineral metabolism, healthy bones and nervous system, muscle tone, reproductive health, insulin production, protection against depression, and protection against chronic diseases like cancer and heart disease.

Vitamin K plays an important role in growth and skeletal development, normal reproduction, development of healthy bones and teeth, protection against calcification and inflammation of the arteries, myelin synthesis and learning capacity.

Vitamins A, D and K work synergistically. Vitamins A and D tell cells to make certain proteins; after the cellular enzymes make these proteins, they are activated by vitamin K. This synergy explains reports of toxicity from taking vitamins A, D or K in isolation and why taking whole food sources are better that isolated supplements. All three of these nutrients must come together in the diet or the the body will develop deficiencies of the missing activators.

The vital roles of these fat-soluble vitamins and the high levels found in the diets of healthy traditional peoples confirm the importance of pasture-feeding livestock. If domestic animals are not consuming green grass, vitamins A and K will be largely missing from their fat, organ meats, butterfat and egg yolks; if the animals are not raised in the sunlight, vitamin D will be largely missing from these foods.

Consumed in liberal amounts during pregnancy, lactation and the period of growth, these nutrients ensure the optimal physical and mental development of children; consumed by adults, these nutrients protect against acute and chronic disease.

Vitamins A, D, and K2 for a Straight Spine

BONE DEVELOPMENT

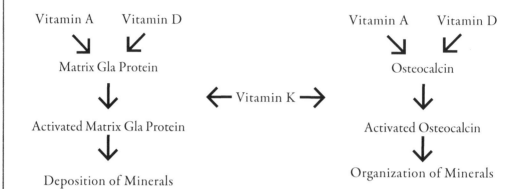

Vitamin A   Vitamin D   Vitamin A   Vitamin D

Matrix Gla Protein   ← Vitamin K →   Osteocalcin

Activated Matrix Gla Protein   Activated Osteocalcin

Deposition of Minerals   Organization of Minerals

BONE GROWTH

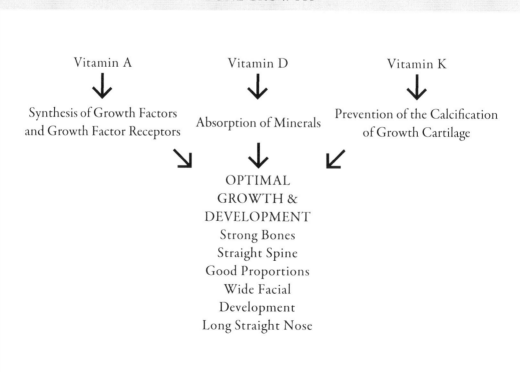

Vitamin A   Vitamin D   Vitamin K

Synthesis of Growth Factors and Growth Factor Receptors   Absorption of Minerals   Prevention of the Calcification of Growth Cartilage

OPTIMAL
GROWTH &
DEVELOPMENT
Strong Bones
Straight Spine
Good Proportions
Wide Facial
Development
Long Straight Nose

Sources of Fat Soluble Vitamins

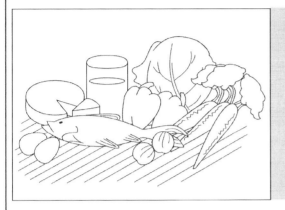

Vitamin A

Vitamin A is found in animal sources like beef/calf liver, fatty fish (mackerel), cod liver oil, egg yolk and dairy products. Beta-carotene, a precursor to vitamin A, is found in green leafy vegetables, and brightly colored fruits and vegetables.

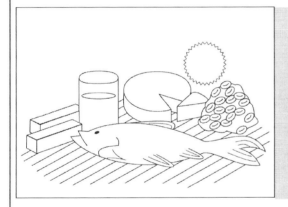

Vitamin D

Vitamin D is made by the body when exposed to the sun. Foods such as cheese, butter, milk, cod liver oil and fatty fish (mackerel, sardines and herring).

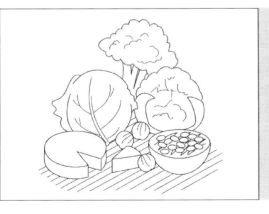

Vitamin K

Vitamin K is manufactured by the beneficial bacteria in your intestines hence fermented foods and drinks such as natto and kefir are good sources. Food sources of vitamin K include cabbage, cauliflower, spinach, broccoli, green leafy vegetables and cheese.

CHAPTER 11

Nutrients for Bone and Joint Health

"The doctor of the future will no longer treat the human frame with drugs, but rather will cure and prevent disease with nutrition."

— *Thomas Edison*

E very day it seems we are getting bombarded by ridiculous claims about some new diet, supplements, pills or programs promising us the sun, stars and eternity but often delivering nothing more than dust.

It's understandable if you're skeptical, but you surely do deserve to know how the plan and all the information included in this book will truly improve your health and life.

To begin with, it is important to know that you do not need to consume a shopping bag full of supplements, because the healthy recipes and foods recommended in health books will typically provide you with most of the nutrients you need, provided you are sticking to making food choices based on your particular Metabolic Type®.

The only exceptions may be:

- The few supplements that nearly everyone needs such as fish oil with omega-3, and
- Specific supplementation for those with special health challenges.

The Truth about Supplements

You may be surprised to know that China is actually one of the largest exporters of many drugs and vitamins. About 90 percent of all vitamin C sold in the United States comes from China. They also produce 50 percent of the world's aspirin and 35 percent of all Tylenol. The same holds true for the export of vitamins A, B-12 and E.

Hot on the heels of the poisoned pet food scandal, milk and reported instances of toxic food and toothpaste, all eyes are now turning toward the Chinese vitamin and supplement market, casting doubt on their safety.

Thus, although supplements can sometimes be helpful, your best bet would be to try to derive a majority of your vitamins and minerals from the food you eat. Processed foods are sorely lacking in nutrients, but eating plenty of raw organic foods, farmed locally (or as nearby as possible) and fermented foods covered in the previous sections of this book, can fulfill a majority of your nutritional needs.

New research suggests that oranges provide better antioxidant protection than vitamin C tablets. Fruits rich in vitamin C are powerful antioxidants that can protect cellular DNA from damage.

A research team gave test subjects a glass of blood-orange juice and another group an equivalent amount of vitamin-C-fortified water or sugar water (containing no vitamin C). Blood plasma vitamin C levels shot up dramatically for both the groups of subjects who drank juice and the fortified water, but when their blood samples were later exposed to hydrogen peroxide, a substance known to cause DNA damage, the damage was significantly less in the samples taken from those who drank natural orange juice!

In fruit, vitamin C exists in a matrix of other beneficial substances, which may all interact with each other to produce beneficial effects. Nature is infinitely more complex and intelligent than anything packaged in a product manufactured by the human mind and laboratory.

One common misconception about nutrition is thinking that you only have to pop one multivitamin tablet a day, and then you're set for the rest of the day. People think, "OK, I've covered all my vitamins and minerals for the day because I took this one pill, and that's it." This does not go very far, though, because even though multivitamin pills may be helping you in some small way, they don't provide sufficient nutrition for peak health or disease prevention and, in the process, miss a lot of nutrients not yet discovered. **Hence for optimal supplementation avoid synthetic isolates altogether and, if you must, consume only whole foods or supplements derived from those natural foods.**

My Opinion on Supplements

Some people think that being healthy requires spending a fortune on herbs and supplements, but that's not the case. Although supplementation is one of the strategies put forth here, it doesn't cost as much as you might think if you're smart about where you get your nutritional supplements. By and large, many of these health habits are both highly effective and most importantly most are free of charge. The five habits of health transformation are what I consider to be the five most effective strategies in this quadrant. They are as follows:

1. Sunshine
2. Water
3. Stress reduction
4. Physical exercise
5. Natural whole foods

Recommended Supplements for Scoliosis

1. Whole Food Multivitamins

When it comes to synthetic multivitamins, busloads of research exists — research that details how your body can only absorb a small percentage of the nutrients (and potentially use even less). It's also obvious from this research that your body will absorb greater amounts of nutrients if the multivitamin comes in a non-synthetic natural whole food form.

So, in recommending a high-quality multivitamin, remember that these nutritional supplements complement the food you eat. They do not take the place of a healthy diet of unprocessed organic foods.

Your busy schedule may prevent you from cooking healthy whole food and cause you to eat more "fast food," but this can be detrimental to you and your family's health in the long run. A number of carefully controlled studies indicate that by the time such "fast" food reaches your table, serious nutrient content is already lost. Some estimate this to be as much as 50%!

The loss could partly be attributed to conventional farming methods that rely heavily on the use of chemical fertilizers and pesticides. In other cases, cooking can also rob food of its nutritional value. So, realizing that you cannot always obtain the whole unprocessed foods you need — and knowing how easy it is for valuable nutrients to be destroyed — you now know why adding a good **whole-food based** multivitamin to complement your diet is a sound decision.

2. Bone Broth

Have you heard the South American proverb, "Good broth can resurrect the dead."?

Nothing can beat the goodness of homemade broth — rich, fragrant, and glistening with droplets of golden fat! Homemade bone broth offers such depth of flavor that its store-bought variant can never parallel. You can use it as a base for soups, sauces, gravies, as well as providing a cooking medium for grains and vegetables.

As the bones cook in water — especially if that water has been made slightly acidic with cider vinegar — minerals and other nutrients get released from the bones into the water, turning it rich with calcium, magnesium, phosphorus and other trace minerals. What's more, bone broth even contains glucosamine and chondroitin that help counter arthritis and joint pain. Best of all, homemade bone broths are rich in gelatin, an inexpensive source of supplementary protein.

What Is Broth Made Of?

The two important components of homemade bone broth are proline and glycine, both of which play a very significant role in bone formation. Bone is made of collagenous fibers built from gigantic protein molecules containing some 1,000 amino acids each. Glycine contributes one-third of the total aminos. The other aminos that figure prominently in bone are proline and hydroxyproline.[63]

Here is a brief discussion of proline and glycine:

Proline

Recent research shows that plasma levels fall by 20 to 30% when person of average health is put on proline-deficient diet.[64] This implies that proline should be classified as an "essential" amino acid. The body cannot produce proline in sufficient quantities without dietary assistance.

Glycine

The human body requires huge quantities of glycine for detoxification after an exposure to chemicals. Glycine also helps digestion by enhancing gastric acid secretion.

What Is The Best, Natural Source Of Proline And Glycine?

Research indicates that gelatin is the best source of proline and hydroxyproline, known to man. It contains nearly 15.5 and 13.3 grams per 100 grams of proline and hydroxyproline, respectively. In addition, it also contains 27.2 grams of glycine per 100 grams pure protein. Lysine and hydroxylysine needed for collagen synthesis are also present, albeit in smaller amounts of 4.4 and 0.8 grams per 100 grams pure protein.

Would you believe it? A 1907 Italian study showed that gelatin injections could increase calcium in the circulating blood, thereby stimulating bone building.[65] Recent studies continue to support this effect. In a Japanese study, for instance, a control group of mice was fed for ten weeks with a low-protein diet containing 10% casein, while the experimental group was fed a combination of 6% casein and 4% gelatin. The result?

Bone mineral content and bone mineral density of the femur were both significantly higher in the experimental group than in the control group."[66] And this effect was more pronounced than that experienced with proline, except when the two are used in combination, as a 1999 German study shows.[67]

Likewise, in 2000, while reviewing literature on collagen hydrolysate in the treatment of osteoporosis and osteoarthritis, Dr. Roland W. Moskowitz of Case Reserve University discovered that 10 grams of pharmaceutical grade collagen hydrolysate per day were enough to reduce pain in patients with osteoarthritis of the knee or hip and — this is most important — gelatin held a significant treatment advantage over the placebo.[68]

Convinced? Let's proceed.

The only thing to bear in mind is that whatever form of gelatin you ultimately use, it should NEVER be cooked by a microwave oven. According to a letter published in The Lancet, heating gelatine in a microwave oven converts l-proline to d-proline,[69] which can be hazardous. In other words, the gelatin in homemade broth can confers wonderous benefits, but if you heat it in the microwave oven, it becomes toxic to the liver, kidneys and the nervous system.

The Role of Gelatin in Promoting Gut and Bone Health

Many popular health writers, including Adelle Davis and Linda Clark, have identified severe bone-related problems caused by widespread hydrochloric acid deficiencies, especially after the age of 40. As Davis put it, "Too little hydrochloric acid impairs protein digestion and vitamin C absorption, allows the B vitamins to be destroyed and prevents minerals from reaching the blood to the extent that anemia can develop and bones crumble."[70]

Another researcher, Carl Voit, found that gelatin helps digestion because of its ability to normalize cases of both hydrochloric acid deficiencies and excesses, and belong to that class of "peptogenic" substances that favor the flow of gastric juices in the gut, thereby promoting digestion.[71]

Gelatin's traditional reputation as a health restorer has hinged primarily on its ability to soothe the GI tract. "Gelatin lines the mucous membrane of the intestinal tract and guards against further injurious action on the part of the ingesta," wrote Erich Cohn of the Medical Polyclinic of the University of Bonn back in 1905.

Likewise, Dr. F M Pottenger found that if gelatin is included as part of the meal, digestive action is distributed throughout the mass of food and digestion of all components proceeds smoothly.[72]

Gelatin and the Liver

Reuben Ottenberg, M.D. wrote in the Journal of the American Medical Association: "It has been suggested that the administration of extra amounts of proteins containing an abundance of glycine (such as gelatin) can improve liver metabolism."[73] Ottenberg recommends that patients with jaundice and other liver problems take 5 to 10 grams of gelatin per day either in the form of food or as a powdered medicinal supplement.

In Summary…

Bone broth is a perfect antidote for people with scoliosis and also in the following conditions: arthritis, inflammatory bowel disease (Crohn's disease and ulcerative colitis), cancer, decreased immune system states, and malnutrition. Gelatin is the key ingredient in broth, although it also contains several other nutrients and minerals (e.g. calcium, phosphorus, magnesium, sodium, potassium, sulfate and fluoride) essential for bone and gut health.

Think of bone as a protein and a calcium supplement. The chemical ingredients extracted from broth are glycine and proline (collagen/ gelatin), calcium and phosphorus (minerals), hyaluronic acid and chondroitin sulfate (GAGs), and other minerals, amino acids and GAGs in smaller amounts. The All New Joy of Cooking describes broth as inherently calming, consoling, and restorative to our spirit and vigor.[74]

I recommend the use of bone broth in soups on a regular basis during all stages of scoliosis and most importantly during a child's growth spurt. While traditionally, soup is served at lunch or dinner, I highly recommend it for breakfast too because it has a high water and mineral content which is ideal in the morning, when your body is dehydrated and fasting from several hours of sleep. You can use the bone broth to make any soup you like so long as you make sure you follow the instructions below.

How to Make Your Own Bone Broth At Home

Key ingredients

1. Bones — from poultry, fish, shellfish, beef, lamb

- Cooked remnants of a previous meal, with or without skin and meat
- Raw bones, with or without skin and meat
- Use a whole carcass or just parts (good choices include feet, ribs, necks and knuckles)
- Don't forget shellfish shells, whole fish carcasses (with heads) or small dried shrimp

2. Water — start with cold filtered water

- Enough to just cover the bones
- Or 2 cups water per 1 pound bones

3. Vinegar — apple cider, red or white wine, rice, balsamic

- A splash
- Two tablespoons per 1 quart water or 2 pounds bones
- Lemon juice may be substituted for vinegar (citric acid instead of acetic acid)

4. Vegetables (optional) — peelings and scraps like ends, tops and skins or entire vegetable

- Celery, carrots, onions, garlic and parsley are the most traditionally used, but any will do
- Remember if you add these towards the end of cooking, the mineral content in the broth would be higher

Method

Throw in the coarsely smashed pieces of bones, water and vinegar into a pot, let stand for 30 minutes to 1 hour. Then bring this water to a simmer, remove any scum that has risen to the top, reduce the heat, cover, and simmer (6-48 hrs for chicken, 12-72 hrs for beef) again. If desired, add vegetables in the last ½ hour of cooking. Strain and discard the bones. Cold broth will gel when sufficient gelatin is present. Broth may be frozen for months or can be refrigerated for about five days without spoiling.

3. Sunshine and Health

A Chinese or an Indian would find it hard to believe that a new California law bans kids under the age of 14 from getting "fake bakes", and that in 27 US states, teens need their parent's permission to tan outdoors! The concern stems from the fact that over-exposure to the sun can allow ultraviolet (UV) rays to invade our skin, resulting in damage to the DNA and eventually leading to skin cancer.

If you recall what I mentioned in an earlier part of this book, one man's food can be another man's poison, and vice versa. Alarming reports of the harmful effects of too much sun on our skin and bodies is propagated by the Western media because their fair skin does not carry enough pigmentation (melatonin) to protect them against the harmful effect of the ultra violet light present in the sun's rays.

In contrast, the same sunlight can be life sustaining for darker-skinned Afro-Asians. It's not without reason that some ancient Eastern civilizations declared that "the sun feeds the muscles."

Even the Romans followed a training practice of sunbathing their gladiators in order to strengthen and enlarge their fighting muscles. Olympian athletes also took sunbaths and along the Bay of Gascony, people still believe that sunlight cures rheumatism. Many people who suffer from arthritis pain state that they feel much less pain during the summer than they do in the winter if they happen to live in countries with a harsh winter climate.

My own personal belief in the matter is that there is perhaps not a cell in our body that does not directly or indirectly benefit from sun light. Just as plants would be unable to do any photosynthesis and survive without sun, human beings also need sunlight to synthesize new life.

Adventurer Dan Buettner visited four spots on the globe where people lived well into their 90s and 100s and painstakingly analyzes how they add years of good life in his book, *The Blue Zones*.

After visiting these places, the author came to the conclusion that exposure to sun — a source of vitamin D — is common in "blue zones" where the longest living societies exist.

In one section of the book Buettner writes, "We shouldn't be burning ourselves, we shouldn't be frying. But 20 minutes a day, in the climates or the latitudes that have quality sunshine, it's probably a good takeaway."

Vitamin D is a Key Player in Your Overall Health

It bears emphasizing that Vitamin D, once linked only to bone diseases such as rickets and osteoporosis, is now recognized as a major player in overall human health.

In a paper published in the December 2008 issue of the *American Journal of Clinical Nutrition*, Anthony Norman, an international expert on vitamin D, identifies vitamin D's potential contribution to good health in the adaptive and innate immune systems, the secretion and regulation of insulin by the pancreas, heart and blood pressure regulation, muscle strength and brain activity. Access to adequate amounts of vitamin D is also believed to be beneficial towards reducing the risk of cancer.[75]

Norman also lists 36 organ tissues in the body whose cells respond biologically to vitamin D, including bone marrow, breast, colon, intestine, kidney, lung, prostate, retina, skin, stomach and uterine tissues. All of your body organs and cells have receptors for vitamin D, meaning that vitamin D communicates all around your body. Your cells use vitamin D to directly regulate your genes, making it one of the most powerful compounds in human health. Canada has even made it law in some provinces that all nursing home residents be given supplements of vitamin D!

In a report published on June 19, 2009, in the journal *Osteoporosis International,* the International Osteoporosis Foundation's expert working group on nutrition revealed the global extent of vitamin D insufficiency. They found that suboptimal vitamin D levels are common in most areas of the world, and appear to be on the rise. The authors reviewed published literature concerning the vitamin

D levels of people residing in Asia, Europe, Latin America, the Middle East and Africa, North America and Oceania. What they discovered was that vitamin D deficiency was prevalent in South Asia and the Middle East, where increased urbanization and the wearing of clothing that covers most of the skin are major contributors.

A recent study linking low vitamin D levels to bone disorders has been done by a team of scientists at the All India Institute of Medical Sciences (AIIMS), in New Delhi, India.[76] The research, led by Ravinder Goswami of the department of endocrinology and metabolism at AIIMS, lends credence to the fact that vitamin D deficiency can lead to life-threatening emergencies in young populations that have not developed protective bio-adaptation over time.

After their first systematic study of blood serum in 2000, which showed more than 75% of healthy people studied in northern India had vitamin D deficiency, this group of researchers has shown that though our skin has darkened to adapt to tropical climate, there is no bio-adaptation to this deficiency. In other words, dark skin, which prevents ultraviolet ray mediated vitamin D to be formed in the body, does not lead to over-expression of vitamin D receptor, a hormone that regulates calcium levels in the body.

As a result, researchers say, they suffer from bone disorders like rickets, osteomalacia and osteoporosis, which are widely prevalent in the subtropical countries. Their two new studies were recently published in the *British Journal of Nutrition* and the *European Journal of Clinical Nutrition*.

This study elaborates that in the early stage of vitamin D deficiency, our body adapts by increasing the parathyroid hormone in the blood, which helps in maintaining normal calcium levels and, hence, the deficiency is not easily detectable. In the long run, however, this leads to bone resorption (bone breaks down to release calcium in the blood) and osteoporosis (reduction in bone density, which enhances risks of fracture).

All this calls for a national policy on vitamin D fortification of food, just as is common in the West. The overarching claim for fortification comes from Goswami's other study, which shows that 60,000 units (IU) of vitamin D taken once a week for eight weeks, along with 1g of elemental calcium every day, restored the baseline vitamin D level. However, the levels dropped one year after vitamin D supplements were stopped.

Therefore, direct exposure to sunlight, for at least a half-hour per day, is what researchers suggest for adequate vitamin D intake during the warmer months or sun tanning parlors in the colder months.

The only concern in maintaining an optimum dosage is that too much of a good thing can also be bad. Care must be taken not to burn the body. Too little, rather than too much, should be the rule. Begin the sunbath by exposing the entire body six to ten minutes a day and gradually increase the length of exposure to half an hour or a little more. Expose the front of the body three to five minutes, and then expose the back three to five minutes.

At the beginning of the warm season, begin to go out gradually, perhaps as little as ten minutes a day. Progressively increase your time in the sun so that in a few weeks, you will be able to have adequate sun exposure with little risk of developing skin cancer. Unfortunately chronic levels of vitamin D deficiency cannot be reversed overnight, and it may take months of supplementation and sunlight exposure to rebuild the body's bones and nervous system.

Vitamin D for Your Bones, Joints, and Teeth

When it comes to bone health, vitamin D and calcium go hand in hand, as the former helps in the absorption of the latter. The prevalent dietary calcium intake is 307-340mg in urban populations and 263-280mg in rural populations, which is less than a third of the required calcium (1 gm/day). As a consequence, even though these people live in the sunniest part of the globe, they remain deficient in Vitamin D.

Vitamin D is not only important for bone formation and growth from conception through childhood, but is also necessary for regulating bone-turnover throughout life. It is important for the health of teeth, and increases muscle strength, mass, and coordination.

Diet has a significant impact on how D works in the body. Protein is necessary for bone and muscle mass maintenance, and magnesium, along with omega-3 fats, slow bone turnover. Acidosis-stimulating foods such as cheese, salt, and grains drain calcium, magnesium, and protein from bones and muscles, and work against vitamin D. Green leafy vegetables are essential for bone and muscle health and balancing the acid-base in the body.

With the typical American diet being high in acid-producing foods and low in greens and other vegetables, it is no wonder that the leading cause of disabilities in our population are diseases involving muscle, bone, and joints; lower back pain is the number one cause. Cases of osteoarthritis, gout, and pseudogout, even strength and coordination issues, can all be linked to low levels of vitamin D, and are improved when these levels are raised to within normal ranges.

People experience an increased risk of bone breakage as they grow older, caused by the skeletal disease osteoarthritis. While it affects older generations, the propensity towards developing it is set up early in life. During childhood, the less protein, calcium, magnesium, and phosphorous that is integrated into the skeleton, the higher the risk later in life. As adults, the lower your levels of vitamin D, the higher your risk of fracture due to a lower bone mass. Because of this, it is important to maintain normal levels of D during pregnancy. Children must get enough of the vitamin through sun or supplements as well as in their diet, complete with adequate protein and omega-3s, and parents should ensure their children do plenty of weight-bearing exercises such as climbing trees, playing sports, or riding bicycles to help guarantee healthy bones.

Studies have shown direct connections between cavities, tooth loss, and gum disease and the development of cardiovascular disease and multiple sclerosis. Dental health is a good outside indication of what is going on with the bones on the inside. People who have extensive tooth loss most likely are not only lacking in bone mass, but also are severely deficient in vitamin D as well. Supplementation of vitamin D, along with calcium, can reduce the rate of tooth loss and help bones as well.

Following the recommendations of the vitamin D cure can lower the risk of arthritis by 50 percent, and the same goes for the risk of muscle weakness, loss of coordination, and the falling that is associated with aging. Those with higher vitamin D levels show a 26 percent reduction in osteoporosis, but if diet and vitamin D have been maintained since conception, a 50 percent reduction of risk can be expected.

Even Doctors are Deficient in Vitamin D

Whether people get their vitamin D from sunlight, vitamin supplements, foods rich in vitamin D, or some combination of these sources, there is no good reason for anyone to ignore the body's need for this vital nutrient. Also people shouldn't wait for the doctor to suggest vitamin D levels be tested. As Dr. Michael Hollick, a medical doctor and author of UV Advantage, concluded after conducting a study at the Boston Medical Center in 2002 (as reported by MedicalConsumers.org), 32% of students and doctors between 18 and 29 were found to be vitamin D deficient.

What about Cod Liver Oil?

Cod liver oil is a commonly recommended supplement, due to its richness in vitamins A, D and omega-3. These three nutrients are all necessary for proper growth and development, especially in children.

With further study, it would appear that cod liver oil is not as safe as once thought. Modern processed cod liver oil contains much more vitamin A than vitamin D than is normally found naturally, and for some this may be dangerous, especially as we learn more about how these two vitamins enhance the activity of each other.

New studies have shown that not only are both of these vitamins important, but the ratio of these vitamins to each other is crucial. Taking in too much vitamin A can sabotage the benefits realized from adequate intake of vitamin D; however, if you take in too little vitamin A, vitamin D cannot fulfill its potential either. Too much or too little of either vitamin can affect the balance of the other.

Most cod liver oil produced today does not supply these vitamins in proper ratio to each other. Unfortunately, we do not know what the best ratio between the two should be, and manufacturers seem to add or subtract these vitamins at will or whim.

Two studies help to shed light on this theory. The first showed that people who supplemented vitamin A in the form of cod liver oil actually were 16% more likely to die than people who did not. The second showed that vitamin A supplementation in developed countries (such as the U.S.) did not decrease their risk of infection. They actually increased their risk!

This is where the issue of correct ratios comes into play. In third world countries, people obtain most of their nutrients from grains, and thus are largely vitamin A deficient. In developed countries such as the U.S., this is not the case; in fact, approximately 5% of people in the U.S. have vitamin A toxicity.

A Harvard researcher conducting studies into reducing the risk of colon cancer found that people who had high levels of vitamin A and vitamin D did not enjoy higher levels of protection against colon cancer. In fact, those with normal levels of both vitamins had a reduced risk of colon cancer. This led him to believe that those who did not supplement with vitamin A enjoyed the positive effect of higher levels of vitamin D.

Researchers believe that when you supplement with vitamin A, you effectively inhibit vitamin D from bonding to your DNA in its active form, thus preventing vitamin D from regulating the expression of your genes.

To clarify, it is the retinol form of vitamin A that is problematic. Beta carotene poses no risk because it is pre-vitamin A, and your body will only convert what it needs as long as you're healthy enough. If you are deficient in vitamin D and supplement with retinoic acid, you are more likely to build up toxic levels of vitamin A which can result in liver damage.

The best way to obtain the necessary ratio of vitamin A to vitamin D is naturally. Vitamin A can be obtained in the diet, through adequate intake of colorful vegetables, and vitamin D through daily sun exposure on your skin. If this is not possible because you're stuck in an office or school all day, then supplementing with Vitamin D3 would suffice. If you would still like to supplement with cod liver oil, then visit the Weston A. Price Foundation website (www.westonaprice.org), for a list of recommended brands of cod liver oil.

Supplementing with Vitamin D3

It is widely recognized that vitamin D levels are low in many individuals in our modern society where a majority of the population is indoors for most of the day. It is due to this fact that supplemental Vitamin D3 maybe a convenient alternative to getting direct sunlight. The American Government, for example, recommends levels of vitamin D dietary intake from 400 IU to 600 IU per day, which most likely is insufficient based on a significant body of vitamin D science. Many vitamin D researchers believe that 2000 IU are needed on a daily basis, especially in the winter months. Vitamin D intake of 2000 IU has been safely tested in children ages 10-17. In fact, only the dose of 2000 IU was able to bring the common vitamin D deficiency in children up to normal levels.

In a study of overweight African-American children, it was found that 57% who were overweight lacked vitamin D, compared to 40% of the control group. However, 1 month of vitamin D intake at 400 IU per day failed to bring vitamin D levels into normal range, indicating that current government recommendations are inadequate.

A new study with young healthy men found that they needed 700 - 800 IU of vitamin D per day in the winter to maintain optimal bone health. You can imagine that the elderly, most women, or individuals with a health condition such as scoliosis would need a higher amount.

In my view, part of the issue of how much Vitamin D you need should be based on clinical tests or on the symptoms you have that indicate likely deficiency. How much vitamin D is optimal? There is no way to know for certain, and the answer may be dependent on several factors, such as:

As a general rule, older people need more vitamin D than younger people, bigger people more than smaller, heavier people more

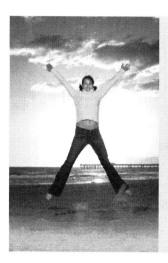

- ☐ age
- ☐ body weight
- ☐ percentage of body fat
- ☐ latitude (where you live)
- ☐ skin coloration
- ☐ season of the year (summer versus winter)
- ☐ use of sun blocking agents
- ☐ how much sunlight you are exposed to regularly
- ☐ your health status

than lighter, northern people more than southern dwellers, dark-skinned people more than lighter-skinned people, sun block users more than those who shun its use, and ill people more than those who are in good health.

As you can see, there are multiple factors involved in how much vitamin D each individual needs. There is no strict formula, and the need for vitamin D can change according to the individual's health status. If you become ill and suffer from heart disease, cancer or even scoliosis, how much vitamin D will your body require to help you become well? No one knows the answer to this question, but based on the most recent large-scale clinical research findings I recommend the following ranges:

Reference Ranges for Vitamin D levels

Deficient	Optimal	Treat Cancers	Excess
< 50 ng/ml	50 – 65 ng/ml	65 – 90 ng/ml	>100 ng/ml

Testing Vitamin D Levels

Before considering supplementation with vitamin D, it would be wise to have your vitamin D level tested. This is best done from a nutritionally oriented physician. It is very important that they order the correct test, as there are two vitamin D tests — 1,25(OH)D and 25(OH)D.

25(OH)D is the better marker of overall D status. It is this marker that is most strongly associated with overall health.

The correct test is 25(OH)D, also called 25-hydroxyvitamin D.

If you have the above test performed, please recognize that many commercial labs are using the older, dated reference ranges.[77] The above values are the most recent ones based on large-scale clinical research findings. For safety purposes it is advisable to optimize your vitamin D levels only with the help of a trained health care professional. Ideally, the best place to get vitamin D is from your skin being exposed to the UV-B that is in normal sunlight.

4. Omega-3

One nutrient which is essential for health is omega-3 which tends to be severely lacking in modern everyday foods. Omega-3 fatty acids are essential fatty acids, necessary from conception through pregnancy and infancy and, undoubtedly, throughout life.

Generally our diet contains far too much omega-6 fats. Experts looking at the dietary ratio of omega-6 to omega-3 fatty acids suggest that in early human history the ratio was about 1:1. Currently, most people eat a dietary ratio that falls between 20:1 and 50:1. The optimal ratio is most likely closer to the original ratio of 1:1. For most of us this means greatly reducing the omega-6 fatty acids we consume and increasing the amount of omega-3 fatty acids.

There are three types of omega-3 fatty acids:

- Alpha-linolenic acid (ALA) [NOTE: ALA is also commonly used as the acronym for Alpha Lipoic Acid — not the same thing.]
- Eicosapentaenoic acid (EPA)
- Docosahexaenoic acid (DHA)

ALA is available from certain plants, such as flax seeds, walnuts and a few other foods, but the more beneficial omega-3s, EPA and DHA, must be obtained from marine sources.

Modern-day families generally consume low levels of omega-3s, a fat primarily found in fish oil (and a few other foods). Meanwhile, our intake of omega-6 is too high. This fat is common in corn, soy, sunflower, margarine and other vegetable oils too commonly used today. Acceptable oils include high-quality extra virgin olive oil, coconut oil, avocados and organic butter, or better yet grass-fed organic butter.

Another way to improve your omega-6 to omega-3 ratio is to change the type of meat you are eating. Since nearly all cattle are grain-fed, making them high in omega-6, if you eat most traditionally-raised supermarket beef, it will typically worsen your omega 6: omega 3 ratio.

Grass fed beef tends to have the same ratio of Omega 6:3 as fish, with a 6:3 ratio of 0.16 to 1. This is the ratio science suggests is ideal for our diet.

Omega-3 fatty acids are essential to strengthen cell membranes of tissues found in the retina, brain, and sperm and act to prevent disease throughout the body and spine. Omega-3:

- Fights spinal conditions such as rheumatoid arthritis, ankylosing spondylitis and scoliosis,
- Maintains normal heart function,
- Has anti-inflammatory properties,
- Helps with normal growth and development of the nervous system,
- Balances cholesterol,
- Improves the immune system.

5. Probiotics

Did you know that:

- About 80% of your immune system resides in your gastrointestinal tract.
- 500 species of bacteria live inside you.
- About one hundred trillion bacteria live inside you — more than TEN TIMES the number of cells you have in your entire body.
- The weight of these bacteria constitutes about two to three pounds.

We discussed it in an earlier section, but there is no harm in reiterating that some bacteria found in our body are actually good for our health. The ideal balance between good and bad bacteria should be 85% good to 15% bad bacteria.

Probiotics increase the amount of good bacteria in our body. When ingested, these living micro-organisms replenish the micro flora in our intestinal tract. This kind of replenishment can result in a number of health-sustaining functions, including enhanced digestive support.

Historically, people used fermented foods like yogurt and sauerkraut as food preservatives to limit spoilage, and to support their intestinal and overall health. In ancient India, it was commonplace (as is still a practice) to have a yogurt-based drink called *lassi,* before every meal. Again, at the end of the meal, they consume a small serving of curd. These ancient traditions were based on the principle of using sour milk as a probiotic delivery system.

Likewise, the Bulgarians are noted for their longevity and their high consumption of fermented milk and *kefir.* In Asian cultures, pickled fermentations of cabbage, turnips, eggplant, cucumbers, onions, squash, and carrots are still common. I often wonder how or why we discontinued those good practices and under whose influence?

The processed foods so inherent in our modern-day diets can upset the balance of good bacteria. Further, many food products are pasteurized or sterilized and if nothing else, these processes destroy and kill all bacteria, thereby eliminating the good bacteria that is normally found in fermented or cultured foods.

I don't advise people to buy the premium-priced, sugar-packed 'health drinks' which claim to contain beneficial bacteria — their high sugar content (some brands contain more per weight than cola!) depletes any probiotic level. I do, however, recommend that you top off your levels with a good quality probiotic supplement if you're too busy to make your own fermented foods.

Since good bacteria are increasingly being missed in our modern diets, it's essential to supplement our food with probiotics. This gives the GI tract and the immune system an extra "edge" — to maximize the benefits of a healthy diet.

Kefir And Vegetable Culture Starter

If you are serious about boosting your immunity and increasing your daily energy, then adding traditionally fermented foods to your diet is a must. Although not widely known, the health benefits of these foods are tremendous.

Tryptophan, one of the essential amino acids found in kefir, is well known for its relaxing effect on a strained nervous system. Because it also offers large amounts of calcium and magnesium — both of which are critical to the nervous system — kefir in the diet can have a particularly calming effect on the nerves.

As discussed in a previous section, kefir is rich in vitamin B12, B1, and vitamin K and is an excellent source of biotin, a B vitamin which aids the body's absorption of other B vitamins, such as folic acid, pantothenic acid, and B12. The many advantages of maintaining adequate B vitamin intake range from regulation of the normal function of the kidneys, liver and nervous system to helping promote healthy looking skin, boosting energy and promoting longevity.

Cultured food was a healthy mainstay in the diets of our ancestors. Only a minimal portion of their foods were even cooked — raw foods, full of live enzymes, made up the majority of their diet. The "modern" methods of pasteurization and adding chemicals to speed fermentation of products like yogurt and cheese have killed these once enzyme-rich foods and converted them to poisons that disable our digestion and ultimately endanger our health.

Cultured foods help reestablish the natural balance of our digestive system. Through the ancient art of fermentation, these foods are partially digested by friendly enzymes, fungi, and good bacteria — making their nutrients readily available to your body. In addition to enhanced flavor and nutrition, cultured foods also offer a multitude of medicinal rewards. When you eat raw cultured vegetables loaded with enzymes, you give your body an opportunity to make enzymes to rejuvenate itself, instead of wasting a large portion of your enzymes digesting food.

You can easily make cultured vegetables by shredding cabbage or a combination of cabbage and other vegetables and then packing them tightly into an airtight container —leaving them to ferment at room temperature for several days. During fermentation, the

friendly bacteria are rapidly reproduced to convert sugars and starches to lactic acid.

Once the initial process is over, you can slow down the bacterial activity by putting the cultured veggies in the refrigerator.

The cold greatly reduces the fermentation, but will not stop it completely. Even if the veggies sit in your refrigerator for months, they will not spoil; instead they become more appetizing over time — much like a fine wine.

In addition, the beneficial bacteria naturally present in the vegetables promptly lowers the pH, making a more acidic environment so the bacteria can reproduce. The vegetables become soft, tasty, and slightly "pickled." The enzymes in cultured vegetables also help digest other foods eaten with them, aiding in the breakdown of both carbohydrates and proteins.

Now these traditionally fermented products are easier to make with the use of "culture starters" which contain a variety of bacteria designed for either kefir or vegetable ferments. I highly recommend these starters to ensure that your milk or vegetables begin fermenting with a hardy strain of beneficial bacteria, which also eliminate toxic components from food and destroy a number of potential pathogens during the fermentation.

6. Vitamin K2: The Forgotten Vitamin

Vitamin K has been shown to:

- Prevent conditions of the bones from developing, such as scoliosis and osteoporosis
- Help in preventing damage to the joints and cartilage and could possibly prevent and treat osteoarthritis[78]
- Serve as a binding agent for calcium and bone matrix, "gluing" them together
- Act as both a preventative and a treatment in certain cancers[79]
- Help in preventing atherosclerosis (hardening of the arteries) and, by extension, coronary artery disease and heart attacks[80]
- Aid in improving memory

Vitamin K is unlike other vitamins. It does not build up to toxic levels in the body (you can't get "too much" vitamin K), and it acts similarly to a hormone. Vitamin K is a potent antioxidant and can help reduce the signs of aging.

What is the recommended dosage of vitamin K? The jury is still out, but the research on this important vitamin is still ongoing so the daily recommended amount is still unknown. What is known, however, is that most adults have some degree of deficiency. Studies show that children are more likely to be deficient because they are still growing. In fact, recent recommendations have been issued that state newborn infants should receive an intramuscular injection of vitamin K at birth to prevent vitamin K deficiency. Vitamin K doesn't cross the placenta very well, leaving most infants deficient in this important vitamin. The injections help to promote proper bone development and to prevent bleeding due to the fact that vitamin K helps your blood naturally clot.[81]

Also, those with intestinal dysfunction may be deficient due to the fact that their digestive flora produces inadequate amounts of vitamin K.

What are the best sources of vitamin K? Dark green leafy vegetables are one source, as is grass-fed animal fat. Natto, cheese and goose liver are also rich in vitamin K.

Those who wish to supplement vitamin K2, in order to treat a condition or because they do not have easy access to foods rich in vitamin K, will find that there are two forms available:

- MK-4 (menaquinone-4) — a synthetic supplement which is less expensive than MK-7
- MK-7 (menaquinone-7) — a natto extract

No studies have compared the two, therefore it cannot be concluded that one is better than the other, but choosing a natural extract over a synthetic supplement is generally a better choice.

A word of caution: Vitamin K is known to interfere with the blood-thinning properties of warfarin (Coumadin). Patients taking this medication should only supplement with vitamin K on the advice of their physician.

All forms of vitamin K are fat-soluble; therefore, in order for your body to absorb vitamin K, you should consume some fat with it. A good place to start is a dose of 45 mg per day as research shows an increase in bone mineral density.[82] To experience further benefits for bone and vascular health, 100 mg per day of supplemental Vitamin K2 is suggested.

Part 3

Corrective Exercises for Scoliosis

CHAPTER 12

How Your Spine Works

"An ounce of action is worth a ton of theory."

— Friedrich Engels

Before sharing with you some of the major tools that will help you design a personalized exercise/fitness therapy that is uniquely suited to the specific condition of your spine, let me first explain in this section how our spine works.

- A spine that is afflicted by scoliosis will understandably look different in its outward appearance, and will also function differently from a normal spine, both aspects of which we will cover in this section.

- In addition, I will also explain to you about the role of the vertebrae, intervertebral discs, spinal cord, sacrum, pelvis and muscles in keeping your spine normally aligned.

- Finally, with the help of detailed illustrations, I will explain spinal biomechanics, that is, how your spine functions and regenerates. Last but not the least, the importance of exercise and good body mechanics to bone health in both pre- and post-scoliosis surgical patients.

Remember that my goal here is to help improve your back posture, foster aerobic fitness, maximize range of motion and strength, and clarify ways in which you can successfully manage your scoliosis. The exercise program that I have outlined in this part of the book will eventually assist in calming your pain and inflammation and improve your mobility and strength, besides helping you carry on with your day-to-day activities like a completely normal person. Therapeutic exercises, such as those outlined in this book, can help maximize patients' physical abilities, including flexibility, stabilization, coordination, and fitness conditioning. In general, this program incorporates the following set of exercises:

Flexibility

Flexibility exercises are helpful in creating safe movement. Tight muscles cause imbalances in spinal movements, thereby causing injury. Gentle stretching increases flexibility, eases pain, and reduces the chance of re-injury.

Stabilization

The "core" muscles you'll be working on are closer to the centre of the body and act as stabilizers. These key muscles are trained to help position the spine safely and to hold the spine steady as routine activities are performed. These muscles form a stable platform that let the limbs move with precision. If the stabilizers aren't doing their job, the spine may be overstressed with daily activities.

Coordination

Strong muscles need to be coordinated. As the strength of the spinal muscles increases, it becomes important to train these muscles to work together. Learning any physical activity takes practice. Muscles must be trained so that the physical activity is under control. Spine muscles that are trained to control safe movement help reduce the chance of re-injury.

Fitness Conditioning

Improving overall fitness levels aids in recovery from spine problems. Fitness conditioning involves safe forms of aerobic exercise, including swimming laps, walking on a treadmill, using a cross country ski machine, or using a stair stepper.

Functional Training

Chiropractors often use functional training when patients need help doing specific activities with greater ease and safety. Examples include posture, body mechanics, and ergonomics.

Posture

Being careful about your posture can reduce strain on the joints and soft tissues around the spine. As strength and control are gained with stabilization exercises, proper posture and body alignment will be easier to remember and apply in all activities.

Body Mechanics

Daily tasks, such as getting out of a chair, pulling yourself out of bed, taking out the trash, hanging clothes on the line to dry and brushing one's teeth, should all come easily and smoothly with an understanding of body mechanics.

Ergonomics

Even minor changes in the furniture you use; the chair you sit on, the angle of an arm rest, and the direction of the bed you sleep on can go a long way in sorting problems related to scoliosis. All this comes under a new branch of science called ergonomics.

To understand how scoliosis causes the spine to curve to the left or right, you need to first understand what a normal spine looks like.

To begin with, there are four regions in your spine:

Anatomy of Your Spine

Cervical Spine: This is your neck, which begins at the base of your skull. It contains 7 small bones (vertebrae), which doctors label C1 to C7 (the 'C' means cervical). The numbers 1 to 7 indicate the level of the vertebrae. C1 is closest to the skull, while C7 is closest to the chest.

Thoracic Spine: Your mid-back has 12 vertebrae that are labeled T1 to T12 (the 'T' means thoracic). Vertebrae in your thoracic spine connect to your ribs, making this part of your spine relatively stiff and stable. Your thoracic spine doesn't move as much as the other regions of your spine, like the cervical spine.

Lumbar Spine: In your lower back, you have 5 vertebrae that are labeled L1 to L5 (the 'L' means lumbar). These vertebrae are your largest and strongest vertebrae, responsible for carrying a lot of your body's weight. The lumbar vertebrae are also your last "true" vertebrae; down from this region, your vertebrae are fused. In fact, L5 may even be fused with part of your sacrum.

Sacrum and Coccyx: The sacrum has 5 vertebrae that usually fuse by adulthood to form one bone; the coccyx (most commonly known as your tail bone), has 4 (but sometimes 5) fused vertebrae.

Your spinal column, also called your vertebral column, has 24 individual bones — your vertebrae. In between the vertebrae, you have intervertebral discs that act like pads or shock absorbers. Each disc is made up of a tire-like outer band (annulus fibrosus) and a gel-like inner substance (nucleus pulposus).

Together, the vertebrae and the discs provide a protective tunnel (spinal canal) for the spinal cord and spinal nerves. The spinal cord runs from the brain down through most of the spine. Nerves branch off the spinal cord at intervals and exit through openings called the foramen. From there, nerves go to various parts of your

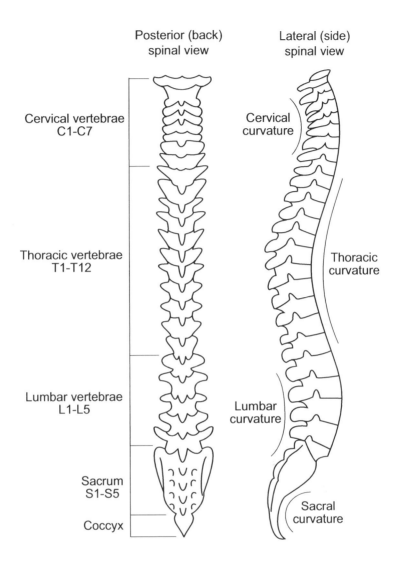

Figure 9: Anatomy of the spine.

body, helping you move and feel sensations such as heat, cold, pain, and pressure.

In addition to bones, nerves, and the discs which cushion and protect these bones, your spine is also supported by ligaments and muscles.

Muscle and Ligament Changes in Scoliosis

The action performed by muscles is to contract; in other words, muscles can pull in one direction only. If you think of muscles as ropes, it is easy to envision what your muscles are capable of: if you pull on a rope, the rope is strong and can support great amounts of weight; however, if you try to push on a rope it will simply buckle. Muscles have the remarkable ability to respond to stress by contracting or stretching. In the scoliotic spine, the muscles on the concave side of the curve tend to be shortened, while the muscles on the convex side are stretched.

While no two scoliosis are the same, so too are the differing muscles that work on the spine to give it its unique appearance. In the examples shown in Figure 10 and 11, it shows the interaction of various hypertonic (overactive) muscles that play a role in

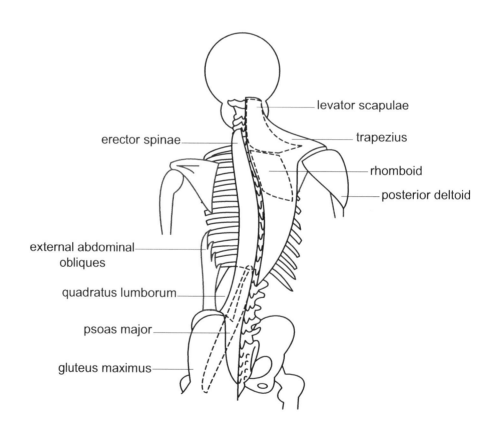

Figure 10: Muscles that tend to be hypertonic for a C-shaped scoliosis

differently shaped curvatures. For example, Figure 10 illustrates a C-shaped curve to the right. It can be seen that the rhomboids, trapezius, posterior deltoid, and levator scapulae muscles act on the spine, pulling it to the right. The left erector, psoas, quadrates lumborum, and gluteal muscles act on the bottom half of the spine to pull it back into midline position. The action (and opposing actions) of the muscles give the spine the C-shape that characterizes this form of scoliosis.

Figure 11, on the other hand, illustrates an S-shaped scoliosis. An S-shaped scoliosis involves more muscle groups because there are, in essence, two separate curves. You can see that different muscles will be involved depending on the direction of the curve(s) and the position of the curve in the spine (i.e. upper or lower back).

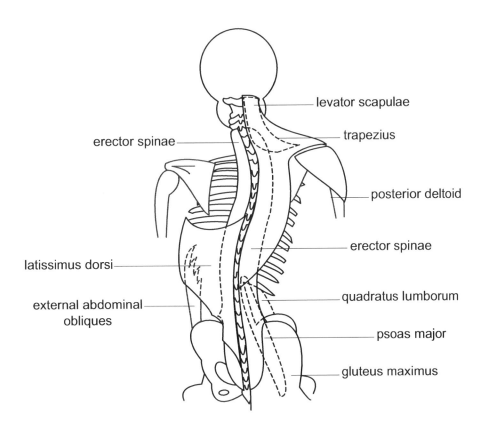

Figure 11: Muscles that tend to be hypertonic for a S-shaped scoliosis

Where do ligaments fit in? First of all, it is important to understand what ligaments are, and what purpose they serve.

Ligaments are connective tissues that hold bones together, forming a joint. They are composed of fibrous tissue, which has "give," or the ability to stretch. They help to control how much movement a joint has, as well as stabilizing the joint so that bones are not able to move too far out of proper alignment.

Ligaments will generally be tight on the concave side of the scoliosis, and less so on the convex side of the curve. Ligaments play a very important role in stabilizing the spine. Together with your muscles, your ligaments work to hold your spine in a relatively straight position. If you have scoliosis, these ligaments and muscles must work twice as hard to do their job, which can lead to back pain and strain.

Mapping Your Scoliosis

To be able to correct your scoliosis, you need to first figure out which muscles feel tight and which are stretched out. Following is an example of a person's back with their S-shaped scoliosis fully mapped out with muscle tightness and locations of the spinal curvature (Fig. 12). Follow the steps below to map out your own scoliosis on Figure 13 and to understand your body more closely.

This is how you should proceed:

First draw in your scoliosis — based on your latest X-rays — onto Figure 13. If you don't have an X-ray report, get another person to run his/her finger down your spine feeling for the spinous processes (the bumps that go down your back).

Next map out the areas of muscle tightness with an **XXX**. For assistance, refer to Figures 10 and 11 for the typical muscle tightness's are usually present for a S or C shaped scoliosis.

Figure 13 will be important in designing your own exercise program for your spine.

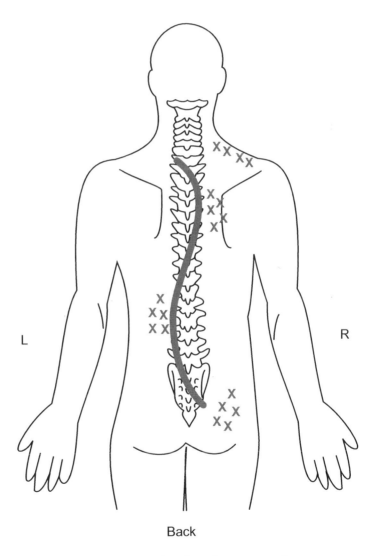

Figure 12: Example of Scoliosis Map showing where the person feels tightness.

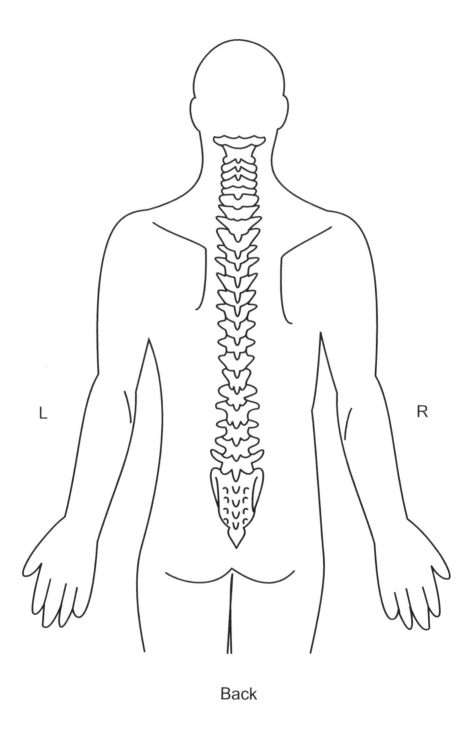

L　　　　　　　　　　　R

Back

Figure 13: Using the diagram map your Scoliosis

Mapping the Symptoms of Your Scoliosis

In order to be able to correct your scoliosis, it is necessary to determine which muscles are affected, and identify the areas of your back where you most often experience symptoms such as pain, numbness or pins and needles. Refer to the diagrams provided in this book.

You will be able to refer back to these diagrams later on; I strongly believe that if you follow a diet suited to your Metabolic Type® and follow an exercise program according to the principles outlined in this book, one day you will be free from the pain and discomfort that currently plagues you.

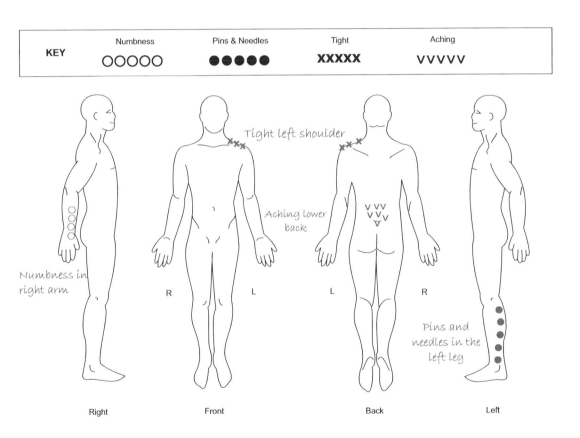

Figure 14: Example of mapping out your symptoms

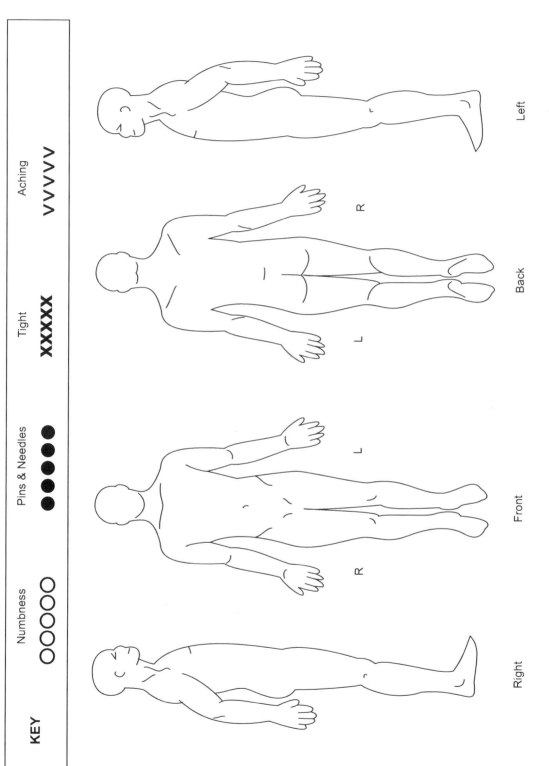

Figure 15: Using the diagram provided map out your symptoms.

Can Exercise Help My Scoliosis?

The answer is a resounding "yes!" I have seen it in my practice time after time: strengthening and stretching play an important role in the correction of scoliosis. In 2008, a comprehensive literature review of 19 papers, which included 1,654 treated patients and 688 controls, revealed that "all studies confirmed the efficacy of exercises in reducing the progression rate (mainly in early puberty) and/or improving the Cobb angles (around the end of growth). Exercises were also shown to be effective in reducing brace prescription."[83]

Over the last five years, eight more papers from throughout the world (Asia, United States, and Eastern Europe) have been published, all attesting to the value of exercise in treating scoliosis, and showing that interest in exercises to treat scoliosis is not exclusive to Western Europe. These studies confirm and strengthen the previous ones. The evidence gathered by the studies to date show that exercise for adolescent idiopathic scoliosis is helpful not only in the prevention of scoliosis, but also its correction!

Reversing Spinal Degeneration or Injury

The prevailing myth is that once spinal damage has occurred, including disc and nerve damage, you either need surgery or are condemned to live with the pain, weakness and other organ malfunction for the rest of your life.

This cannot be farther from the truth. By following some of the tips shared in this book and by incorporating a regular exercise plan in to your life, you cannot only heal your spine, but sometimes even reverse the process of spinal damage. How do the intervertebral discs rehydrate and regenerate? The spinal discs need three things to regenerate: motion, water and nutrients. It is a well-known, scientific fact that an upright, adult spine loses up to 20 mm of vertical height each day due to loss of fluid from the disc. During sleep some of this fluid and the consequent height are regained, but not all, with the result that by the time a person turns 60, he/she can end up losing quite a bit of this disc fluid and bone flexibility. Indeed, a loss of just 12 percent of the water out of the discs can reduce disc height by as much as 50 percent!

Since almost 88 percent of the disc composition is water, proper hydration is essential for nourishment, lubrication and function of all joint cartilages, tendons, ligaments and spinal discs' nutrition delivery and waste elimination.

However, as people get older, they often become more sedentary, developing advancing spinal and postural degenerative conditions and ultimately losing some portion of the natural flexibility in their spine. That's when the discs begin to dehydrate and lose height. This is the main reason why chronic lower back pain tends to occur when someone is sitting for long periods of time rather than walking or exercising. When a person is sitting in front of the computer or TV for an extended period of time, the spinal discs dehydrate, leading to the holes where the nerves exit from the spine to get smaller and eventually become pinched. When this happens, chronic pain begins to occur that soon advances to more serious loss of muscle function and sensation, depending on what that particular nerve it happens to be associated with at that particular spinal level.

Research has shown, if we can create loading and unloading cycles in our spine, we can actually "suck" water back into the disc and rehydrate it predictably. Loading and unloading cycles are nothing more than consecutive alternating compression and traction movements as the spine is going through motion. Simply put — your spine thrives on physical activities whether that be walking or swimming.

If you start early, when the spine is young, supple and flexible and the effects of scoliosis are not too far advanced, the results can be more rewarding. Done with the right nutrients and exercises recommended in this book, it would very soon be possible for you to re-generate your spine and introduce some degree of correction and healing.

Case Study: Taking Control of Your Spine

Cher's parents discovered she was "limping" when she was thirteen and worried. They noticed that her left leg was shorter than her right. On the advice of a senior nurse, who was a family friend, the adolescent was taken to a doctor who diagnosed it as scoliosis. This was the first time, her parents heard about the disorder. She had a 38 degree C shape curve in the lumbar area. Her back was cast in a hard plastic body brace all day long. It helped the back problem, but caused another — it seriously dented the teenager's self confidence. She hated the brace and the restrictions it imposed on her lifestyle and the choice of dresses that she could wear. She had to don a school uniform that was at least two sizes bigger than her normal size and it looked completely atrocious on her! Stung with her classmates' barbs, she slowly began retreating into her shell. She became extremely shy and withdrawn.

Worse, she couldn't do even half the exercises that her physical education teacher asked for as doing them gave her bruises from the rough edges of the brace. She had to carry two school bags. It took three to five hours each day to-and-fro school, and she still remembers the shame of walking in the hot afternoon sun with her body soaking wet inside the hard brace. As years went by, she learnt to live with the crooked spine — to pick clothes that could disguise her unsymmetrical body and gave up hope of ever getting treated.

In April 2006, she had a serious backache and was bedridden for almost a week. She was deciding to relocate to Australia when her sister brought her a newspaper clipping about my seminar. After researching on the internet, she decided to postpone her relocation plan and give my treatment a try.

The pre-treatment X-ray showed that her curve had indeed worsened over the years, to 55 degrees, and was affecting other areas such as her neck. For the next half a year, despite her office work load, she didn't miss a single session with me. The initial treatment was uncomfortable, but two months later her body began to adjust to all the pulling and stretching. Gamely, she went along with it, and gradually her body has begun to yield and turn more flexible. She has started feeling more energetic.

At the end of the six month's treatment, her post-treatment X-ray revealed a 15 degrees improvement in her scoliosis. At the end of therapy, she told me that her dad had been taking photos of her back with the digital camera and even he could tell the difference.

"To me, the whole experience of the treatments meant much more than the 15 degrees of correction in my spine. I felt that in many ways I was blessed, and I learnt to have faith that there is a solution somewhere for any problem."

— *Cher C. (33 year old)*

CHAPTER 13

Posture Retraining

"Posture is the key to life."

— *Mark Twain*

I was once approached by a very concerned father who said: "Dr. Lau, my 14-year-old girl has been diagnosed with scoliosis. The doctors say nothing can be done. We have to 'watch and wait,' and later, maybe consider surgery if the curve in her back increases. She experiences pain and we wonder what would be the best thing for her. Can you help?"

The first thing I told them was that they must stop waiting and watching. That indeed is the worst thing to do. Instead they must act as responsible parents, and act fast. Later, I sat them down and told them the story of evolution.

I tried to explain to them in a manner that they would understand that when our predecessors walked on all fours, their abdominal and thoracic (chest) organs hung from the spine. The spine in that case was supported by their fore and hind legs.

However, as man started to stand and walk upright, his hind legs became a strong support system for the rest of the body, and that's when everything changed. Now the spine had all the organs in front of it, so there was a potential threat of falling forwards. Therefore, over the course of evolution, the muscles of the back developed to compensate, acting like pulleys to keep the spine upright. Today, the spine acts principally as a structure that provides surfaces for muscles to attach to. When the spine twists, curves or bends, the movement is brought about by muscle contraction.

These same muscles of the spine can go into spasm as a result of poor posture, trauma at birth or later in life due to a sedentary lifestyle, chronic one-sided back pain, nutritional imbalances, mineral deficiencies, genetic problems, malformation of the hip joint, and several other factors.

I also explained to them that scoliosis often begins as a spasm of muscles on one side of the spine. This impels the spine to curve to that side, as a consequence of which the ligaments and muscles harden and the spine becomes crooked. Finally, the 'S'-shape curve develops when another group of back muscles in the lower region on the opposite side go into a spasm. The upper curve and the lower curve gradually begin to push against each other, thus relentlessly deforming the spine.

All this implies that the sooner you treat scoliosis, the better it will be. Thankfully, the parents of that little girl understood that the 'watch and wait' approach was not ideal and started her treatment immediately, without further ado.

Scoliosis, Posture and Body Alignment

Poor posture was once thought to be an important contributing factor in the development of scoliosis in the early 19th century. In the U.S., posture training was considered very important in the treatment for the disorder. It fell out of favor only when bracing and surgery became more popular.

From my experience in practice, I have come to understand the importance of postural correction for a scoliotic person. I constantly stress the importance of proper posture and body alignment to my patients, similar to the methods described in antique medical books. Today, we have new names for these age-old techniques: "ergonomics" and "body alignment," but the basic premise remains the same.

Some scientific studies that testify to a strong link between scoliosis and posture include:

- Tethering the spine to one side causes scoliosis[84] in rabbits.
- In a study in Russia, biofeedback was used to correct postural defects[85] and straighten spinal columns.
- A 1979 study in Poland found that posture training and exercise therapy had a role in scoliosis prevention and treatment.[86]
- A 2001 study from Hong Kong showed promising results in scoliosis treatment using posture training.[87] According to the study authors, "A long-lasting active spinal control could be achieved through the patient's own spinal muscles."
- According to a paper in the medical journal *Spine*, studies in Japan and in Sweden have suggested that a disturbance of postural equilibrium exists in idiopathic scoliosis.[88] With this in mind, then it is not surprising that the studies listed above from Russia, Poland and Hong Kong showed positive results on scoliosis curves from posture correction.

When all is said and done, good posture does keep muscles in balance and the body well-aligned. Poor posture, in contrast, places abnormal weight on joints and stresses out muscles and tendons, often leading to pain. Additionally, poor posture does not adequately support internal organs, blood circulation is hampered and a dysfunction is created. When poor posture exists, there is always a need for a stretching program to lengthen short muscles and an exercise program to tighten weak/loosened muscles which we will address in the second part of the book.

How Do You Develop Poor Posture?

In reality, there are many factors that can affect posture ranging from daily habits and activities to genetic predisposition and underlying conditions such as scoliosis, osteoporosis, arthritis, or even pain-inducing conditions that cause chronic habitual positions to be assumed by a person.

However, as with most of the information contained in this book, we have to get back to the fundamental. We were hunter-gatherers evolved to spend our days wandering and doing physical activities such as searching for berries or pursuit of prey and we are no longer doing what we evolved to do. We were not designed to spend our day sitting on our bottoms staring fixedly at a screen or a road, or for any of the other activities of our modern life that are so far from our origins.

Tips on Proper Posture

Good posture is a balanced posture in which positioning is centered so that the pull of gravity is evenly distributed and relaxed for all the joints of the body. With joints in non-awkward positions, muscles relax, and unnecessary tension can be released. Good posture is the most mechanically efficient positioning for the body.

In effect, good posture includes:

- A straight line from your ears, shoulders, hips, knees and ankles
- Head is centered
- Shoulders, hips and knees are of equal height

Some of the most common posture mistakes include:

- Forward Head Lean
- Rounded Shoulders
- Arched Lower Back Or Flat Back
- Excessive Anterior Pelvic Tilt (Protruding backside)
- Excessive Posterior Pelvic Tilt (Protruding abdomen/pelvis)

Test Your Posture

To determine if you have good posture, take the following tests:

The Wall Test

Stand with the back of your head touching the wall and your heels six inches from the baseboard. With your bottom touching the wall, stick your hand between your lower back and the wall, and then between your neck and the wall. If you can get within an inch or two at the lower back and two inches at the neck, you are close to having excellent posture.

The Mirror Test

You can do this simple point check in front of a full-sized mirror, or get your partner or friend to do it for you. Answer these questions and use Figure 16 on the next page to see if:

1. Your head is straight   yes/no
2. Your shoulders are level   yes/no
3. Your hips are level   yes/no
4. Your kneecaps face the front   yes/no
5. Your ankles are straight   yes/no

Now look at yourself from the side (or have someone else check you out) and look for the following:

1. Your head is straight rather   yes/no
   than slumped forwards or backwards
2. Your chin is parallel to the floor   yes/no
3. Your shoulders are in line with ears   yes/no
4. Your knees are straight   yes/no
5. There is a slight forward curve to   yes/no
   your lower back

If you answered "no" to 3 or more of these questions then your posture is not in ideal alignment.

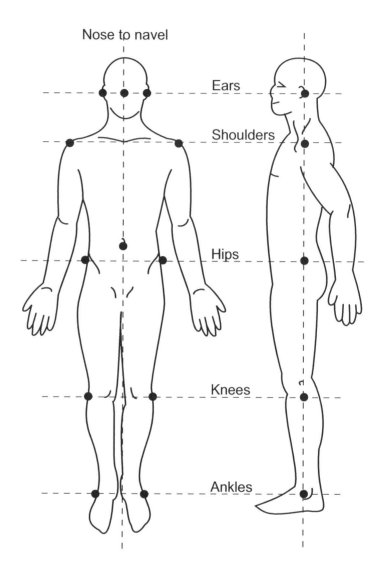

Figure 16: Check your posture in front of a full-size mirror.

How to Correct Poor Posture

Imbalances of body posture can be a sign of imbalance in the spine. Working through the exercises in the following chapters will correct any muscle imbalance you may have and help to establish good posture. Here are two tips to help improve your posture instantly:

1. Imagine you have a balloons attached to the upper part of your chest muscles, and they are lifting them up to the sky. That should immediately improve your hunched shoulders and even the forward head posture. Gently retract your chin, so your neck elongates slightly.

2. Lastly, pull your shoulder blades back toward your spine, and down toward the middle of your back. The reason why you do this is because if you just pull your shoulders back, then you will most likely engage your upper trapezius muscles, which elevate the shoulders. The problem with this is that a majority of people are tight and overworked in these muscles, because this is where they hold their stress. So, we don't want to make them any tighter. Pull the shoulder blades back and down to keep your shoulders relaxed and your chest muscles stretched.

Personal Stories: Law Graduate with Scoliosis

"I was diagnosed with mild scoliosis in 1994. It did not warrant surgery, but it occasionally caused backaches and a slight limp when I walked. In 2005, I heard of a non-surgical treatment that focused on correcting scoliosis. Naturally I was skeptical as this treatment was not well known then. However, a preliminary consultation with Dr. Kevin Lau convinced me that it was a worth a try. Over the course of a few months of regular consultations, my condition steadily improved under his care. His holistic treatment included dietary and lifestyle advice. Some advice seemed radical and hard to accept at the time, but books and newspaper reports soon independently corroborated its efficacy. Dr. Lau's treatment makes his patients centrally responsible for their own wellbeing. So patients who are disciplined, determined and receptive to new ideas stand to benefit most from their time under his care."

— Daryl L. (26 years old)

CHAPTER 14

Body Balancing Stretches

"Life is like riding a bicycle. To keep your balance you must keep moving."

— *Albert Einstein*

Our ancestors led a much more active life than most of us do today. From the Industrial Revolution to present day, machines have taken over more and more of our daily lives. We, in turn, have become much more sedentary. We drive instead of walk, ride the elevator rather than climb stairs, and sit at desks rather than toiling in the fields. As a result, our muscles and bones are weaker and less well-conditioned, and are therefore more prone to injury and disease.

Most of us are aware that exercise is vital to good health. Because we get much less physical activities than in days gone by, it is ever more important that we learn how to stretch properly. Stretching is the bridge between the sedentary world and the active world. One cannot go from being sedentary to being active without crossing this bridge, at least not without risking injury. Stretching keeps your muscles supple, prepare you for movement and help you transition between inactivity and vigorous activity without strain.

Finding Muscle Tightness

Let's begin this section with a self-diagnosis. On Figure 13 in the previous chapter, mark the areas of your back where the muscles are tight i.e. the areas of your back that feel uncomfortable when stretched. To accomplish this, stand up straight with your hands by your side and with straight arms slowly move them in front until they are above your head, keeping your back straight as you do so.

Do you feel some tight spots? Was there any discomfort in your lower back? Was the right side of your lower back tighter than the left? Was your left shoulder more difficult to move than your right? Was there any strain in the back during the movement?

Next, follow the stretching exercises listed at the end of this section concentrating on the spine from your neck to your lower back in the areas that feel the tightest. Repeat each set slowly, while gradually building up the duration of the stretch.

The only way stretching and exercise will be of benefit to you and your condition is if you understand exactly how your body is out of balance. More specifically, you need to know which muscle groups are tight, which muscle groups are weak, and how those imbalances are affecting your body as a whole.

Your primary goal must be to bring your body back to a balanced state in order for your scoliosis to improve. If a muscle group is too strong or too tight and your bones are pulled out of their proper position, eventually your joints will not work correctly. Your joints will suffer wear and tear until eventually all movement will be painful.

There are over 600 muscles that provide mobility to your back, nearly all of them play some role in the health and proper functioning of the spine and all of those muscles need to be exercised on a fairly regular basis.

Also remember that your muscles can pull your pelvis in many different directions. If your pelvis is in an abnormal position such as one side seems to jut out (unlevel), your spine could follow leading to an abnormal curvature. This abnormal curvature will, over time, cause your condition to become painful and gradually become worse.

When all is said and done, irrespective of your age, sex, fitness, or weight, remember we all have imbalances and we all need to understand that stretching and exercise can play a very important role in how we live our lives and how healthy we stay as we grow older. Once you embrace the concept of imbalances, you need to identify where they occur in your body. If you stretch a muscle group that does not need to be stretched, the imbalance is never going to be corrected.

Exercises Precautions

There are some precautions which bear mentioning before you begin to attempt any of the exercises:

- Map out all of your tight and weak muscles before you begin on the diagram provided in this chapter.
- In the manner of an athlete, be absolutely aware which muscles require strengthening and which call for stretching techniques. As a rule of thumb, I suggest practicing the stretches on both sides of the body and making note of which muscles feel tight. Remember: no one is the same and no scoliosis is identical either.
- Practice proper strengthening and stretching techniques as explained in this section, making sure that you feel the targeted areas being worked.

Start incorporating stretches which release tightness in all areas of your spine until both sides feel even and balanced.

Hamstring stretching is also important, as hamstring tightness limits motion in the pelvis. This leads to pelvic imbalance and can increase stress across the lower back. There is a wide variety of ways to do hamstring stretching exercises, including the one mentioned in this book. Find one that you are comfortable with.

Activities like Yoga or Pilates incorporate both stretching and relaxation, which reduces tension in stress-carrying muscles. Yoga requires that the individual hold gentle poses anywhere from 10 to 60 seconds. Within the pose, certain muscles flex, while others stretch, promoting relaxation and flexibility in muscles and joints. Pilates helps with strengthening and shaping the core muscles of your back, abdomen and legs. Both are considered good exercises that keep the spine stabilised and flexible at the same time, and I regularly recommend them for maintenance of the spine after correction. Look out for instructors who are familiar with or specialize in scoliosis.

Any activity that involves excessive jostling or high impact of the spinal column should be avoided. This rules out vigorous sports like cross country running, skiing and horseback riding. Swimming is an excellent physical activity that does, for some patients, ease scoliosis discomfort. While you are in the water, try one of the following:

- Stationary or actual rowing of a boat
- Make bicycling movements with your legs
- Attaching ankle weights while swimming
- Leg lifts while laying on your side and holding on to the side of the pool or a stationary object.

The general recommendation is that you remain physically active every day, exercising aerobically two to three times a week (e.g. brisk walking, cycling, swimming). If you have led a sedentary life, leave a day or two in between your exercise days.

Never over-train. Rest is also an important part of the healing process as this is when muscles and bone heal.

The most widely accepted minimum length of time you should spend exercising is 20 minutes (which does not include the warm-up and cool-down). The maximum is one hour, depending on the exercise you choose. If you are a beginner, try starting with ten minutes.

Correct Stretching Technique

Stretching sounds easy, but when it is done incorrectly, it can lead to injury. It cannot be stressed enough that understanding proper stretching techniques is crucial. Stretching should never be thought of as a contest, and should never be overdone. The goal is not to stretch to the point of pain, but to reduce muscle tension. Stretching should be relaxing and warming, and striving to see who can stretch the farthest should never be a goal—this will lead only to pain and injury. The bottom line is that stretching, when done correctly, should be enjoyable.

In general, choose an exercise plan that is:

1. **Specifically designed for your needs and suits your lifestyle pattern**

   Are you healthy and physically active? Or have you been leading a sedentary lifestyle for the past five years? Are you a professional athlete? Or are you recovering from a serious injury? Do you frequently suffer from aches, pains and muscle and joint stiffness in any area of your body? In all of these scenarios, the exercise plan would have to be different and specially tailored to your needs.

2. **Make a specific review of the area, or muscle group, which needs to be stretched**

Are the muscles ready? Is there any damage to the joints, ligaments, tendons, etc.? Has the area been injured recently, or is it still recovering from an injury?

If the muscle group being stretched isn't 100% healthy, avoid stretching this area altogether. Work on recovery and rehabilitation before moving onto specific stretching exercises.

3. **Don't forget to warm up prior to stretching**

By increasing muscle temperature you are helping to make the muscles loose, supple and pliable. This is essential to ensure that the maximum benefit is gained from your stretching.

4. **Stretch gently and slowly. (Avoid bouncing)**

Stretching slowly and gently helps to relax your muscles, which in turn makes stretching more pleasurable and beneficial. This will also help to avoid muscle tears and strains that can be caused by rapid, jerky movements.

5. **Stretch ONLY to the point of tension**

Stretching is NOT an activity that is meant to be painful; it should be pleasurable, relaxing and very beneficial. Many people believe that they need to be in constant pain to get the most from their stretching. This is one of the greatest mistakes you can make when stretching.

6. Breathe slowly and normally

Many people unconsciously hold their breath while stretching. This causes tension in your muscles, which in turn makes it very difficult to stretch. To avoid this, remember to breathe slowly and deeply during your stretching. This helps to relax your muscles, promotes blood flow and increases the delivery of oxygen and nutrients to your muscles.

The Stretch Reflex

Have you ever touched something hot? Your body automatically, within the blink of an eye, pulls your hand away from the source of the pain without you making a conscious decision. This is an automatic reflex of your nerves in response to a pain stimulus.

Your muscles have a similar reflex, a protective mechanism that prevents them from being harmed inadvertently. When you stretch your muscles too far, the response of your body is to tighten the very muscles you are attempting to stretch!

It is important to listen to your body and pay attention to its signals. When you stretch your muscles excessively, this stretch reflex is activated, and the result is pain. This is your body's way of telling you that you are overdoing it. If you continue to stretch past the point of discomfort, the result is a build-up of scar tissue within your muscles, and a gradual loss of elasticity. If you have scoliosis, damaging the muscles which support your spine is the very last thing that you want to do. Therefore, heed your body's signals and don't over-stretch your muscles.

No Pain, No Gain

Many of us have the idea ingrained in us from an early age that exercise without pain is not beneficial, and that unless we push ourselves to the point of pain, we are not really trying.

This is blatantly incorrect, and can be hazardous. Stretching, when done correctly, should never hurt, but should instead feel pleasurable and relaxing.

Stretch Exercises

In the next section, several stretching exercises that I recommend for my patients with scoliosis are described. Illustrations of the various stretches are also provided to assist you in learning how to correctly perform these stretches.

Many of the stretches described should be held for 20-30 seconds, unless otherwise specified. However, as you become more accustomed to performing these stretches and you become more in tune with your body, you may find that you become more adept at determining just how long you need to hold a stretch to obtain maximum benefit. For example, if you are feeling very limber and are not experiencing any back discomfort from your scoliosis, you may find that holding a stretch for 5-15 seconds is sufficient. On the other hand, if you are feeling very stiff and are experiencing back pain due to your scoliosis, you may need to hold your stretches for longer amounts of time in order to warm up your muscles. Remember: everyone is different and it is important that you listen to your body. Stretch only to the point of feeling tension in your muscles, not to the point of pain.

Neck Side Flexion

Follow the steps outlined below:

- Sit down straight
- You can grasp the end of a bed or the bed for support and then gradually try to lean away until your shoulder is depressed. Make sure that you are maintaining an erect posture, throughout
- Now, use your opposite hand to gently draw your head away from the anchored shoulder
- Inhale and gently push your head into your hand for five seconds
- Exhale and immediately lean further away, while depressing your shoulder. Then gently move your head and neck further away from your shoulder
- Hold the stretch position for 20-30 seconds

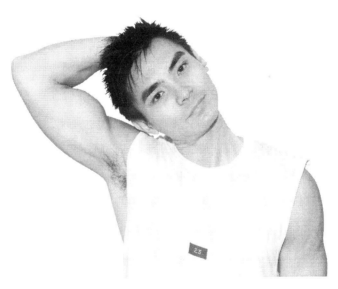

Figure 17: Neck Side Flexion

Neck Rotators

- Sit in a good position
- Rotate your head to one side
- Place the opposite hand on your cheek
- Inhale and gently rotate your head into your hand while keeping the hand firm
- Look in the direction that you are turning
- Hold for 20-30 seconds and exhale as you look behind you and rotate your head into the stretch

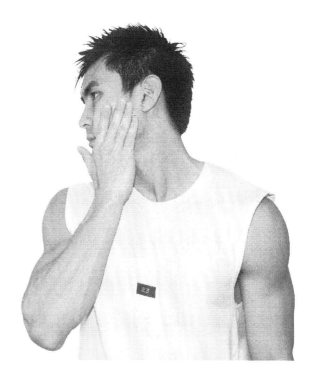

Figure 18: Neck Rotators

Neck Extensors

- Maintain an upright position, either sitting or standing, and let your head drop towards your chest
- Place one hand on the back of your head and one under your chin
- Hold your chin and slightly stretch the back of your neck by drawing your head towards your chest
- Take a deep breath and lightly press your head to your hand, without letting your head move
- After five seconds, relax as you exhale and gently move your head towards your chest

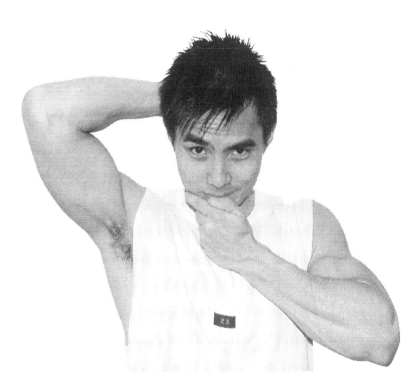

Figure 19: Neck Extensors

Levator Scapulae Stretch

- Place one arm as far down between your shoulder blades as possible
- Look as far as you comfortably can to the opposite side
- Take a deep breath in and hold for five seconds. When you exhale, look downwards as far as you comfortably can towards the shoulder your facing

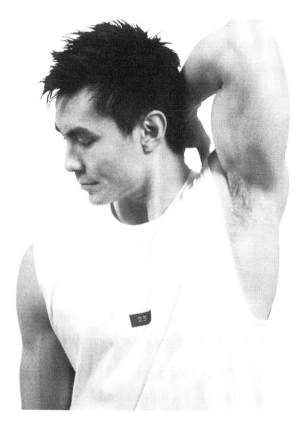

Figure 20: Levator Scapulae Stretch

Scratch Stretch

- Stand with a good posture, holding a towel behind your back as shown in the picture.
- Use the bottom hand to pull downwards until you feel a comfortable stretch
- Hold that position with your lower arm
- Inhale as you try to pull upwards with your top arm against the fixed resistance of the lower arm
- Exhale and pull down with the lower arm to further stretch the upper arm
- **More** emphasis should be placed on the side where the scoliosis making the muscles tighter

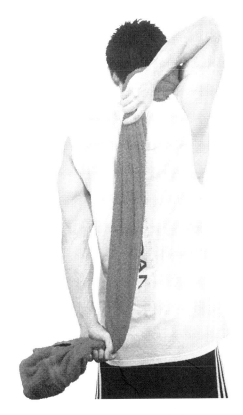

Figure 21: Scratch Stretch

Rhomboids Stretch (between the shoulder blades)

- Kneel with the Swiss ball in front of you and your elbow on the ball
- With the arm resting on the ball bring your arm across your body
- Press the elbow into the ball to stretch the muscles in between the shoulder blade while holding the ball with the other hand
- To increase the stretch, roll the ball with the opposite hand.
- Hold for 20-30 sec

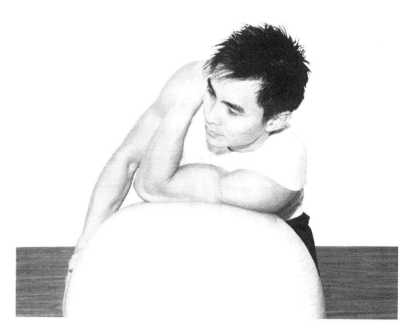

Figure 22: Rhomboids Stretch

Overhead Stretch (hands together)

- In a standing position, feet shoulder width apart
- Extend your arms overhead with your hands together making sure your elbows are straight and thumbs pointing back
- Push your arms back for 20-30 sec

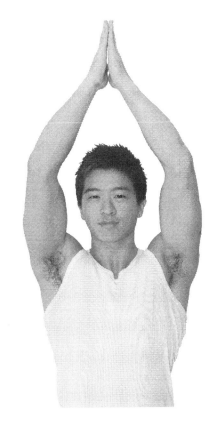

Figure 23: Overhead stretch with hands together

Overhead Stretch (palms inverted)

- In a standing position, feet shoulder width apart
- Invert the hands so that your palms are facing up
- Push your arms back for 20-30 sec

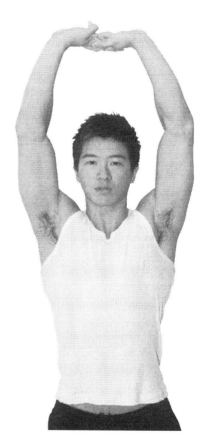

Figure 24: Overhead stretch with palms inverted

Trunk Side Bending (heel sitting)

- In the heel sitting position.
- Lean forward so your abdomen rests on your thighs.
- Stretch both your arms overhead so that's your hands are flat on the floor.
- Then side bend the trunk away from the concavity by walking the hands to the convex side of the curve.
- Hold the position for 20-30 sec for a sustained stretch.

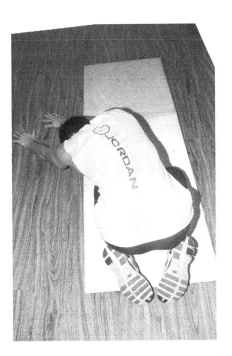

Figure 25: Trunk side bending while kneeling

**Thoracic Side
Bending
(edge of table)**

- Side-lying over the edge of a table
- Place a rolled towel at the apex of the thoracic curve and top arm stretched over head
- With assistance from another person, stabilize the pelvis or lumbar spine for an S curve
- Hold this head/arm down position for as long as possible ~ 1 min gradually increasing up to 5 min

Caution: Due to the hanging position the head is in, stop the stretch if you get dizzy while doing this

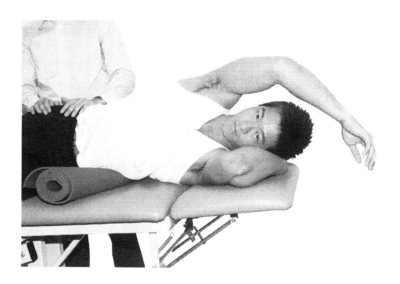

Figure 26: Thoarcic Side Bending (Edge of Table)

Lumbar Side Bending (edge of table)

- Side-lying over the edge of a table with a rolled up towel at the apex of the lumbar curve and top arm stretched over head
- With assistance from another person, stabilize the pelvis
- Hold this head/arm down position for as long as possible ~ 1 min gradually increasing up to 5 min

Caution: Due to the hanging position the head is in, stop the stretch if you get dizzy while doing this

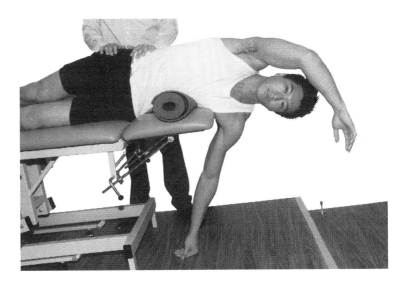

Figure 27: Lumbar Side Bending (Edge of Table)

Lumbar Scoliosis Stretch

- On a table or a mat, lay down on your stomach
- Hold on to the edge of the table, or brace yourself with your arms
- Lift your hips and legs together and with some assistance move them towards the convex side of the curve in the lower back
- Perform a total of 3 times, holding each stretch for 30 seconds

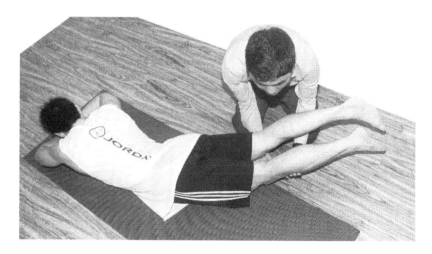

Figure 28: Lumbar Scoliosis Stretch (legs move to the side)

Trunk Rotation

- Lie on your back with your knees bent and pointing up at the ceiling
- Your lower legs should be relaxed. Place your hand on your thigh while keeping the other arm stretched out to help you stabilize
- Slowly let your legs roll to that side until you feel a comfortable stretch in your lower back. Inhale and reduce the support from your arm slightly to activate your trunk muscles
- Hold for 30 seconds and repeat to the other side. Continue to practice this stretch until you can comfortably place your thighs on the ground, or until you are no longer increasing your range of motion

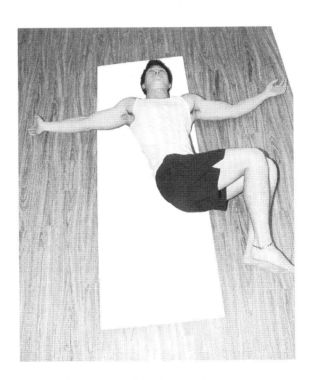

Figure 29: Trunk Rotation

Middle Back and Abdominals

- Be careful to perform this stretch on an anti-skid surface. If you feel any kind of dizziness, stop immediately
- Sit on a Swiss ball, then walk your legs out and roll backwards until you are lying on the ball
- Extend your arms over your head. To increase the stretch, slowly straighten your legs. Hold for one minute

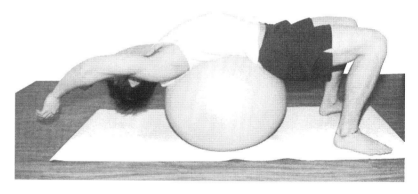

Figure 30: Middle back and abdominals

Hamstrings

- Grab one leg with both hands, just below the knee, and bring the bent leg up until the thigh is perpendicular to the floor.
- Bend your toes back towards your shin and slowly straighten your leg without letting the thigh move in your hands or letting your back come off the floor
- Hold a comfortable stretch for 30 seconds

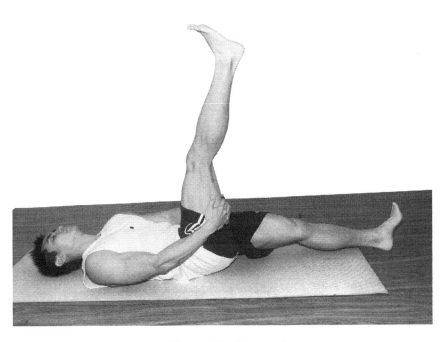

Figure 31: Hamstrings

Iliotibial Band

- Stand next to a wall and step forward with your outer leg, this is the leg that you will be stretching as shown in the adjoining image
- Keep both feet flat on the floor
- Raise your inside arm for support against the wall and place the other hand on your hip
- Press your hip straight towards the wall and slightly downwards as it moves towards the wall
- You should feel a stretch towards the outside of the leg, closest to the wall and in the hip
- If you are performing the stretch correctly, taking your outside hand off the hip at any point will eliminate the stretch in the hip. You should not stretch in your lower back.
- Hold for 30 seconds. Stretch each side up to three times

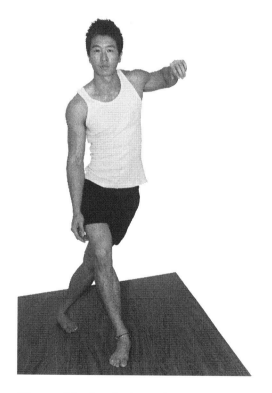

Figure 32: Iliotibial Band outer thigh stretch

Frequently, hamstrings on one side are much tighter than on the other, which can lead to hamstring injuries. Tightness arises because of the presence of a pelvic tilt associated with scoliosis and, on the looser hamstring side, a close-legged, knock-kneed configuration known as jarrete, or hyperextension, causing its own particular difficulties. Consultation with an expert such as a Chiropractor or Physical Therapist is therefore very important before deciding what exercise program to choose for your particular condition.

CHAPTER 15

Building Your Core

"Movement is a medicine for creating change in a person's physical, emotional, and mental states."

— *Carol Welch*

The core that I refer to in this section is your main torso, including your internal organs. Many people believe that the extremities perform most of the hard work and that the core is simply the fulcrum that allows the limbs to move, but in fact the opposite is true: without a strong core, we would be unable to do many of the tasks that we do.

The core is indeed your nucleus, the life force of stability and strength. It's the tree trunk of your body that gives support to the branches, leaves, roots, etc. (Remember the tree analogy that we discussed in Chapter 6.)

The "core" consists of many different muscles that stabilize the spine and pelvis and run the entire length of the torso. The core provides a solid foundation for movement in the extremities. A core conditioning exercise program is thus targeted at these muscle groups that make it possible for you to stand upright and move on your two feet. These muscles help control movements, transfer energy, shift body weight and move in any direction. Needless to say, a strong core distributes the stress of weight-bearing functions evenly, thus protecting the back from injury.

For your spine to be aligned and supported, the muscles forming the core must be balanced to allow the spine to bear large loads.

If you concentrate on strengthening only one set of muscles within the core, you can destabilize your spine by pulling it out of alignment. Think of the spine as a fishing rod supported by muscular guy wires. If all of the wires are tensed equally, the rod stays straight.

Let's take a look at how your core functions in order to appreciate the importance of this area of your body.

The Functions of Core Stabilizers

Support for the Spine

The core is like a corset of muscles and connective tissue that encircle and hold the spine in place. If your core is stable and balanced, your spine remains upright while your body swivels around it and allows the spine to bear large loads.

Protection of Your Central Nervous System and Internal Organs

The core provides a protective shield for your spinal cord and internal organs. The bony spinal column houses the spinal cord, while the rib cage and powerful abdominal muscles act as a shield to protect your internal organs from external blows or invasions.

Support for the Internal Organs

The core houses all the internal organs with the sole exception of vital organs in the head, such as the brain and eyes. When key core muscles stop functioning correctly, support for your internal organs begins to diminish and their function is challenged. This is important for the person who has scoliosis, because as their curve increases, internal organs can become compromised.

Foundation of Movement

The core is your body's foundation for movement. If the core does not function properly, you'll most likely experience extremity and spinal pain, as well as an increased risk of injury.

How to Identify the Core Muscles

The list of muscles that make up the "core" is somewhat arbitrary and different experts group different muscles under this category. The following list includes the most commonly identified core muscles as well as the lesser known groups:

- **Rectus Abdominis** — located along the front of the abdomen, this is the most well-known abdominal muscle group and is often referred to as the "six-pack" due to its appearance in fit and thin individuals.
- **Erector Spinae** — this group of muscles runs along your neck to your lower back.
- **Multifidus** — located under the erector spinae along the vertebral column, these muscles extend and rotate the spine.
- **External Obliques** — located on the side and front of the abdomen.
- **Internal Obliques** — located under the external obliques, running in the opposite direction.
- **Transverse Abdominis (TVA)** — located under the obliques, it is the deepest of the abdominal muscles (muscles of your waist) and wraps around your spine for protection and stability.
- **Gluteus medius and minimus** — located at the side of the hip
- **Gluteus maximus, hamstring group, piriformis** — located in the back of the hip and upper thigh.

A good core exercise program should emphasize all of the major muscles that girdle the spine, including but not concentrating on the abs.

What Disrupts Abdominal Muscle Function?

While there are many reasons why the core stability muscles become weak, I have included three common causes which contribute to the tell-tale "beer belly" or "stomach bloating" that is commonly seen:

1. **Diet/Lifestyle** — consuming foods or drinks that you are allergic to will affect abdominal function. Anything that causes inflammation in an internal organ that communicates through the nervous system and controls an abdominal muscle will cause the muscle to weaken, or be non-responsive to exercises. Other causes of inflammation that can interfere with abdominal muscles are stress, alcohol, medical drugs, food additives, preservatives and artificial food coloring.

2. **Deconditioning** — also called detraining, deconditioning is a term which simply refers to the loss of fitness which occurs due to a decrease in training, or exercising. Many people stop exercising at times for many reasons. Illness, injury, holidays, work, travel and social commitments often interfere with training routines.

3. **Back Pain** — nerves that serve joints of the spine also feed the muscles around the spine. Therefore, anything that causes pain in the spine can upset the muscles and vice versa.

Testing Your Core Processes

There are several exercises available for testing the strength of your abs and building core muscles around your spine. One sports coach, Brian Mackenzie, offers the following core muscle strength and stability test that I have used on myself and with my patients, and that I have found to be pretty effective. The objective of the core muscle strength and stability test is to assess your core strength and endurance over time. It is explained at length in the next few pages.

Before You Begin

To prepare for this assessment you will need:

- A flat surface
- An exercise mat
- A watch or a clock with a second hand for conducting the test

Core Muscle Strength & Stability Test

Level 1: Plank Position

- Start by lying face down on the ground or use an exercise mat. Place your elbows and forearms underneath your chest
- Prop yourself up to form a bridge using your toes and forearms.
- Maintain a flat back and do not allow your hips to sag towards the ground.
- Hold for 60 seconds

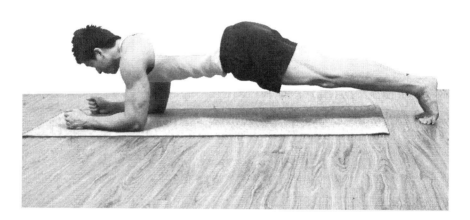

Figure 33: Level 1 - Plank position

Level 2: Plank with Arm Lift

- Lift your right arm off the ground
  Hold for 15 seconds
- Return your right arm to the ground and
  lift the left arm off the ground
- Hold for 15 seconds

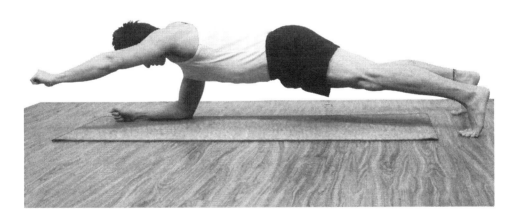

Figure 34: Level 2 - Plank with arm lift

Level 3: Plank with Leg Lift

- Return your left arm to the ground and lift the right leg off the ground
  Hold for 15 seconds
- Return your right leg to the ground and lift the left leg off the ground
- Hold for 15 seconds

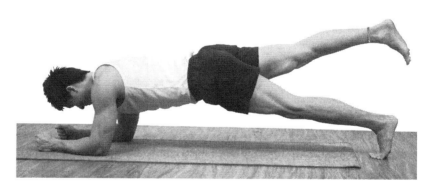

Figure 35: Level 3 - Plank with leg lift

Level 4: Plank with Opposite Leg and Arm Lift

- Lift your left leg and right arm off the ground Hold for 15 seconds
- Return you left leg and right arm to the ground
- Lift your right leg and left arm off the ground Hold for 15 seconds
- Return to the plank exercise position
- Hold this position for 30 seconds

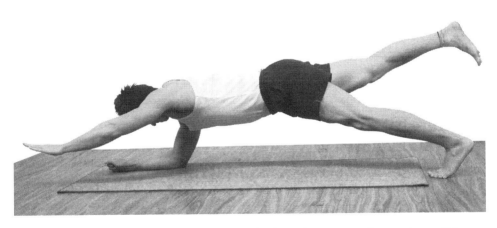

Figure 36: Level 4 - Plank with opposite leg and arm lift

Your Report Card

☐ **Good Core Strength**

If you can complete the test fully, congratulations! You indeed have adequate core stability and are ready to move on to the core stability exercises.

☐ **Poor Core Strength**

If you cannot complete the test fully, your core strength needs improvement. Poor core strength results in unnecessary torso movement and swaying during any vigorous movement. This results in wasted energy and poor biomechanics. Good core strength indicates that you can move with high efficiency, with smooth movements and no muscle tremors.

The Next Plan of Action

If you are unable to complete the test, practice the routine three or four times each week until you improve before moving on to the next level. Master each level of planking until you can complete it comfortably.

By comparing your results over time, you will note improvements or declines in core strength.

Once you are able to complete the core stability test, I recommend that you move on to the beginner and advanced core stability exercises that target different areas of your core.

Before You Begin

What you will need:

- An exercise mat
- A swiss ball (exercise ball)

Beginner Core Stability Exercises

Lower Abdominal Conditioning

- Lie with your back on the ground keeping your knees bent and feet flat on the floor
- Place your hand under your lower back, directly underneath your navel
- Breathe out, draw your navel in toward your spine and gently increase pressure on your hand by flattening the lower back to the ground
- Hold this position as long as is comfortable, up to 10 seconds, then rest for 10 seconds
- Repeat this 10 times
- While performing this exercise, try to relax the entire body while holding the pressure on the hand, focusing on relaxing your jaw, neck, shoulders, trunk and legs

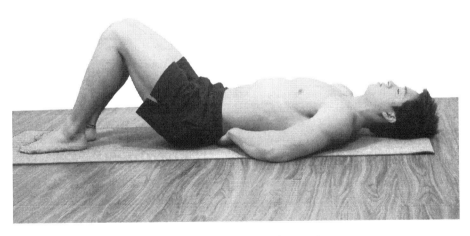

Figure 37: Lower Abdominal Conditioning

Lower Abdominal Conditioning with Leg Lift

- Lie with your back on the ground keeping your knees bent and feet flat on the floor
- Place your hand under your lower back, directly underneath your navel
- Breathe out, draw your navel in toward your spine and gently increase pressure on your hand by flattening the lower back to the ground
- Raise one foot off the ground until your thigh is 90 degrees to floor while maintaining the pressure on the hand
- Place the foot back on the ground and perform the same movement with the other leg
- Alternate legs, performing 10-20 times so long as the pressure on the hand is maintained
- To increase the difficulty, straighten the lifting leg

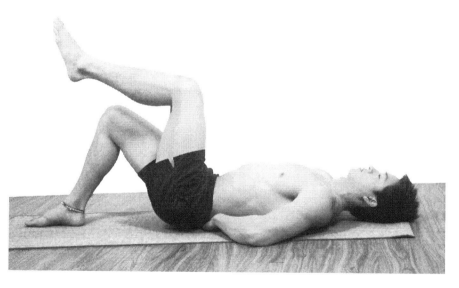

Figure 38: Lower Abdominal Conditioning with Leg Lift

Four-Point Tummy Vacuum

- Kneel down with your hips over your knees and your shoulders over the palm of your hands
- With your spine in a comfortable position without stress in a neutral alignment, take a deep breath in and let your stomach drop toward the floor
- Breathe out and draw your navel in toward your spine, while keeping your back in the starting position
- Hold for as long as you comfortably can
- When you need to breathe in, relax your abdominal wall as you inhale and repeat the exercise 10 times

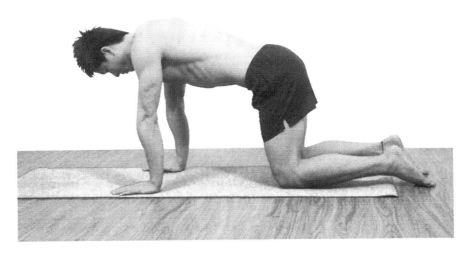

Figure 39: Four-Point Tummy Vacuum

Advanced Core Exercises

Lower Abdominal Conditioning with Double Leg Lift

- Lie with your back on the ground keeping your knees bent and feet flat on the floor
- Place your hand under your lower back, directly underneath your navel
- Breathe out, draw your navel in toward your spine and gently increase pressure on your hand by flattening the lower back to the ground
- Raise both feet off the ground until your thighs are 90 degrees to floor while maintaining the pressure on the hand
- Breathe out and draw your belly button in towards the ground while lowering both legs to the ground
- When it becomes easy to perform the exercise, straighten your legs to increase the difficulty

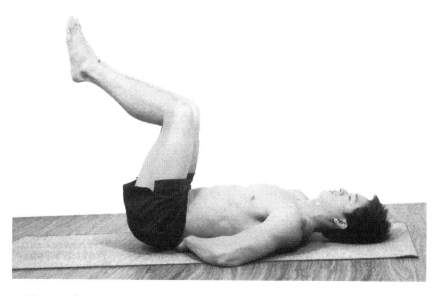

Figure 40: Lower Abdominal Conditioning with Double Leg Lift

Forward Ball Roll

Kneel in front of a Swiss ball with your forearms just behind the highest point of the ball. The angle at your hips and shoulders should be the same. Imagine being able to place a box in between the back of your arms and thighs

- Gently draw the navel inward and hold a good comfortable position of your back and head
- Roll forward, moving your legs and arms in equal measure so that the angles at the shoulders and hips remain equal, as you roll farther away. Progressively increase the effort used to draw your navel inward
- Stop at the point just before you lose form. You will feel your lower back drop down when your form breaks. You should stop just before this point
- For beginners, go to the finish position and hold for three seconds, then return to the start position. Your tempos should be three seconds out, three seconds hold, three seconds return

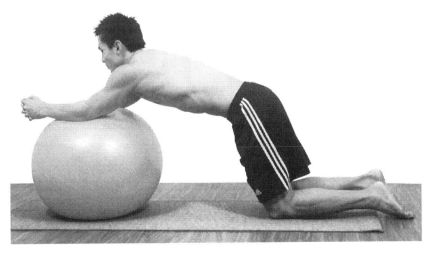

Figure 41: Forward Ball Roll

Jack-knife with Ball

Get into a push-up position with your feet on a Swiss ball and your hands on the floor. Keeping your spine horizontal and knees straight

- Holding your spine in perfect alignment, draw your navel gently in toward your spine. The Swiss ball will roll forward and your knees will come close to touching the ground
- While maintaining neutral spinal alignment throughout the movement, draw your knees towards your chest, hold and then return to the starting position
- Lift your hips as high as needed to bend your knees underneath you, keep your buttocks as low as possible
- This exercise can be made easier by placing the ball closer to your body; for example, on your shins

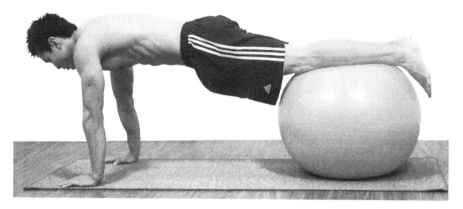

Figure 42: Jack-knife with ball

Swiss Ball Crunch

Caution: If you get dizzy while performing this exercise, you can lean a little forward on the ball In any case, stop this exercise immediately if you continue to feel dizzy

- Lie over a Swiss ball so that your back is comfortably rested on the ball Your head should be extended back and touching the ball
- Keep your tongue against the roof of your mouth
- As you slowly crunch up, imagine that you are rolling your spine from head to pelvis
- On the way back, unwind from the lower back to your head, one vertebra at a time
- Breathe out on the way up and inhale on the way back
- Arm positioning

  Beginner — arms stretched out and reaching forward

  Intermediate — arms kept across chest

  Advanced — finger tips behind ears (do not support your head and neck with your hands)

- **Tempo** — slow, breathing pace
- **Repetitions** — up to 20

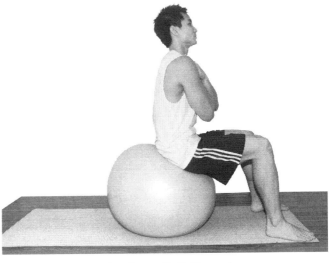

Figure 43: Swiss Ball Crunch —
(A) Beginner, (B) Intermediate, (C) Advanced

Dynamic Horse Stance

- Get on your hands and knees with your wrist directly under the shoulders and knees directly under the hips
- Contract the abdominals and slowly straighten your right leg behind you, turning your foot slightly out while extending your left arm in front of you, thumb up
- Repeat on one side for a set of 10
- Release and repeat with left leg and right arm

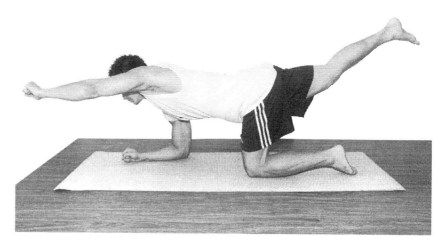

Figure 44: Dynamic Horse Stance

When all is said and done, working on your core is worth the effort. This may be the most significant activity you can do to stabilise, or at least mitigate, the pain of scoliosis. There can be no getting away from the fact that every muscular cause of pain has to be dealt with at the muscular level. Doing these exercises daily will help stabilize your core to give the best support to your spine, as no surgery or brace can do.

Case Study: Setting the Scoliosis Right

Being born with scoliosis, Andrea is now a 44 year old mother of two. The deformity of her spine (i.e. the S-shaped curvature of the spine) was noticed when she was about thirteen years old. Her scoliosis gradually increased as she aged. Breathing was becoming difficult especially after stressful activity, which caused her muscles to pull in her right shoulder and hip. As a result of the scoliotic curve, her body was tilted mainly to the left side and she experienced a creaking in her neck when she attempting to turn her neck. Life was rather difficult to manage and the problem progressed with age.

About 20 years ago, Andrea went to the medical doctor for evaluation on neck pain she was experiencing. At this evaluation, she learned that the curvature of her lower spine had worsened to 45 degrees. She went for a second opinion with another consultant, and was told to wait until the curve had reached 50 degrees to have surgery done. At that time, there were very few treatment options for her.

Recently, Andrea came in to see me and we had her curvature checked. An X-ray showed that her curvature was 55 degrees in the lower spine and about 34 degrees in the upper spine. The curvatures had indeed increased as the years progressed even though she attended standard chiropractic, physiotherapy and yoga sessions during that period.

After a few months of starting the non-surgical scoliosis correction using the methods described in this book, there was an impressive 10 degree reduction in both the upper and lower back giving her a total of 20 degrees correction.

After her non-surgical therapy, Andrea looked much better, and she was very happy with the results. Her breathing problems had reduced considerably and the creaking in her neck, which she experienced often, had also reduced. Most importantly, her body looked more aligned, which improved her physical appearance. She feels more confident now and is doing much better. In the X-rays and photographs of the spine, you can actually notice the difference.

— *Andrea F. (44 years old)*

CHAPTER 16

Body Alignment Exercises

"An ounce of practice is worth more than tons of preaching."

— *Mahatma Gandhi*

I n their book *Backache Relief,* Arthur C. Klein and Dana Sobel[89] surveyed patients with different types of back problems, including scoliosis. At the conclusion of their study, they found that what is most effective for scoliosis patients is not surgery or braces — but prepare yourself for this truth — a regular regimen of exercise! Some experts would like to call it a "functional approach"[90] to the treatment of scoliosis; I prefer to call it the traditional approach to treating scoliosis.

When ligaments weaken and there is degeneration and deformity in the spinal discs and vertebrae, often made worse by the wrong choice of diet, poor biomechanical balance or a sedentary lifestyle, the curved spine can become even worse. In such a scenario, a chiropractor is left with no option but to:

- Detect the deformity at its earliest stage and immediately initiate a process of spinal correction, so that the spine doesn't deteriorate further
- Help you minimize underlying mechanical stresses responsible for the deformed condition of your spine
- Recommend natural ways to strengthen weakened bones, ligaments, and surrounding muscles through an exercise program that is uniquely tailored to your spine condition; and last but not least…
- Regularly monitor the progress made through this exercise program and recommend changes, where needed

Would you believe that in Croatia,[91] physicians continue to advise vigorous sports activities for treatment of scoliosis?

In that region, as in many other places in the world, scoliosis is most commonly found in children who undertake little or no physical activity.

In this context, the Department of Pathology and Molecular Medicine at the Wellington School of Medicine and Health Sciences in New Zealand reports the case of a young boy with progressive juvenile idiopathic scoliosis, who showed remarkable improvement in his spine curvature after undergoing a specifically designed exercise program and physiological traction.

Similarly, doctors at Helsinki University Central Hospital in Finland have found pelvic asymmetry to be an overlooked factor in scoliosis.[92] Their conclusion is that leg-length discrepancies and some neurologic symptoms perpetuate scoliosis. Their usual recommended treatment is also fairly simple, conservative, non-surgical and safe — regular exercise!

As Martha C. Hawes, PhD. writes in her book, *Scoliosis and the Human Spine*, "Statements claiming that scoliosis cannot be stabilized or reversed without bracing or surgery are not, and never have been, supported by scientific data. On the contrary, long-standing basic and clinical research is consistent with the hypothesis that scoliosis can be reduced, if not eliminated using non-surgical approaches."[93]

If more proof is needed that exercise can and does benefit scoliosis patients, here are a few studies that I stumbled upon:

- A spine clinic in San Diego found that out of their 12 patients suffering from adolescent idiopathic scoliosis, four managed to reduce their curves by 20 - 28 degrees after receiving strength training for a certain period of time.[94]

- Almost identical results have been reported from Germany,[95] where bracing with exercise was proven ineffective in conservative scoliosis treatment.[96]
- Another study by a team of chiropractors with a group of 19 patients found that the combined use of spinal manipulation and postural therapy significantly reduced the severity of the Cobb angle in all 19 subjects. One of the methods used in this study was traction.[97]
- Meanwhile, in a study done at the University of Athens, it was found that the ability to perform aerobic work increased 48.1% in patients with idiopathic scoliosis after they received some exercise training, while it decreased 9.2% in the control group.[98]
- Likewise, a paper published in the *Saudi Medical Journal* on the efficacy of Schroth's 3-dimensional exercise therapy for scoliosis patients found that after six weeks, six months and one year of therapy, *all* patients had an increase in muscle strength and recovery of the postural defects. This led the researchers to conclude that the Schroth technique positively influenced the Cobb angle, vital capacity, strength and postural defects in outpatient adolescents.[99]
- Finally as early as 1979, a study in Poland found that postural training and exercise therapy had a definite role in scoliosis prevention and treatment. Another paper from Poland reports positive results from exercise in removing contractures in spinal curvature.[100]

Why Exercise Makes Us Happy!

Research has shown that people who are physically fit are more resistant to spine injuries and pain, and recover more quickly when they do have injuries, than those who are less physically fit.

Indeed, take it from me that any form of exercise, particularly exercise that results in repeated stretching and strengthening of the muscles in your back and neck, are especially beneficial in the treatment of spine-related disorders and can act as powerful relaxants and pain relievers. Sometimes prolonged illness leads not only to physical discomfort but also lack of motivation, but if you can summon the determination to carry on exercising you can successfully address both these problems.

Eventually, a good exercise routine will make the muscles of your back, neck, stomach, and limbs both strong and flexible. After that, it is entirely your responsibility to continue to exercise regularly in order to maintain your current fitness level. That alone will boost your recovery metabolism and give you quick relief from pain and distress.

Just be careful that you do not undertake any strenuous exercise like jogging, jumping, hopping, skipping, marching, tramping, or weight lifting. The use of a sponge rubber cushion while driving or traveling is often recommended to scoliosis patients by orthopaedic specialists.

Before You Begin

What you will need:

- An exercise mat
- A swiss ball
- 2-4kg weights
- Resistance band: light, medium and heavy (depending on your level of fitness)

It takes some time before these exercises can be performed correctly, and a mirror or another person should be used to observe how you perform them.

Neck Exercises with a Swiss Ball

Neck Flexion with Ball

- Stand facing the wall with the ball held on your forehead
- Place your tongue on the roof of your mouth
- Push your head forward into the ball as you exhale
- Repeat 10 times

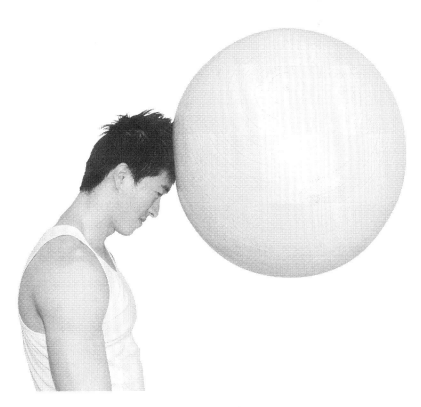

Figure 45: Neck Flexion

Neck Extension with Ball

- Stand with the back of your head against the ball
- You may hold onto a door frame or table for support
- Press your head into the ball as you exhale
- Repeat 10 times

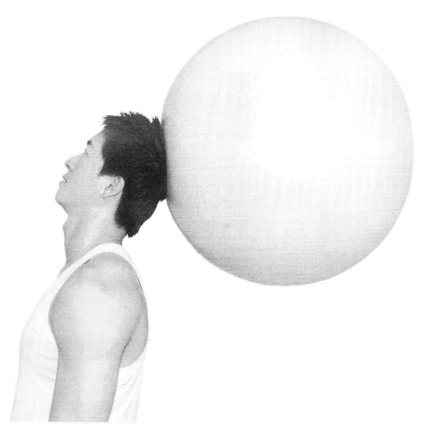

Figure 46: Neck Extension

Neck Side-bend with Ball

- Place the side of your head slightly on the ball
- Bend your neck, pushing your head into the ball as you exhale
- Repeat 10 on both sides. If you have a curvature in the neck, only do this exercise on the concave side

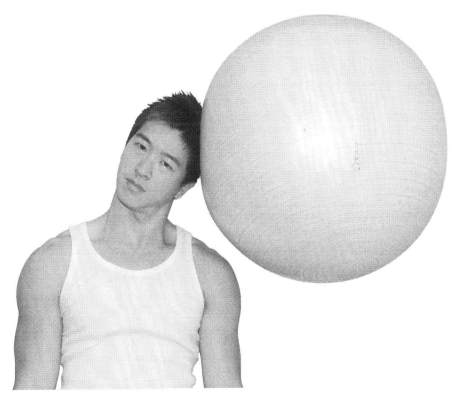

Figure 47: Neck Side-bend

Pelvic Rock Exercises

Pelvic Rock - Front to Back

- Stand with soft knees or sit upright on a Swiss ball
- Inhale and rotate your pelvis forward (imagine that you have headlights on your buttocks and you want to shine the beam upwards.)
- Keep your trunk still as you move your pelvis
- Breathe out and rotate your pelvis back (shine the headlights downwards)
- **Tempo**: breathing pace
- **Repetitions**: 20 each side

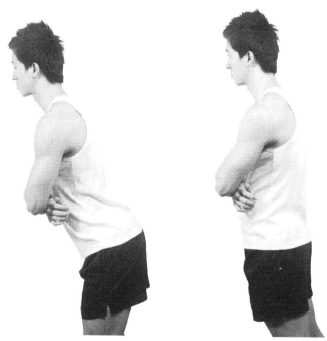

Figure 48: Pelvic Rock Exercise - front to back

Pelvic Rock - Side to Side

- Sit upright on a Swiss ball in a comfortable position
- Inhale and lift one hip up as you breathe out, then return to the start position.
- Inhale and lift the other hip up as you breathe out.
- Repeat going side to side
- **Tempo**: breathing pace
- **Repetitions**: 20 each side

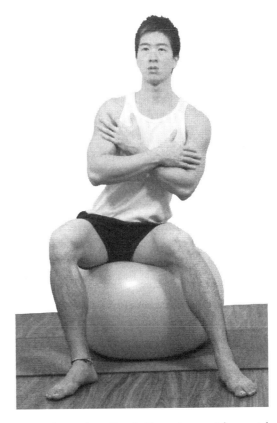

Figure 49: Pelvic Rock Exercises - side to side

Pelvic Rock - Figure Eight

- Complete a figure eight with your hips, moving front to back and then side to side
- **Tempo**: breathing pace
- **Repetitions**: 20 each side

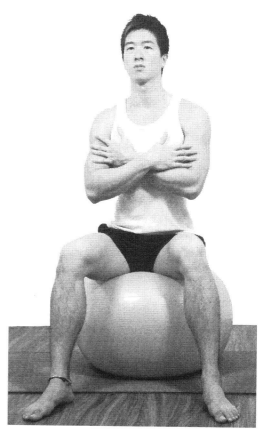

Figure 50: Pelvic Rock Exercises — figure 8

Breathing Squats

If you have lower back pain or experience any discomfort in the breathing squats then use swiss ball squats (fig. 53) as an alternative

- Take a comfortable stance that is wide enough for you to squat down between your legs. Place your arms at your sides or up in front of you for a more advanced version
- Inhale and then lower yourself down as you breathe out. Go as low as you comfortably can, then inhale as you return to standing
- Keep your torso upright and your weight between the balls of your feet and your heels
- The pace at which you lower yourself should perfectly match your breathing rate. Your breathing rhythm should stay the same throughout the exercise. If your breathing speeds up reduce the depth
- **Tempo**: slow
- **Repetitions:** 10

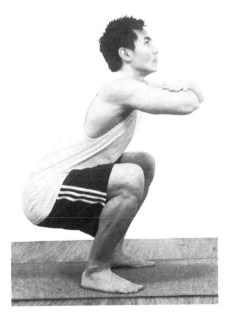

Figure 51: Breathing Squats

Single Arm Overhead Squat

- Take a comfortable stance that is wide enough for you to squat down between your legs. Hold one dumbbell straight above your head
- Inhale and draw your navel inward
- Drop down into a comfortable squat. Keep your torso as vertical as possible. Do not lean to one side
- Breathe out as you return to standing
- Keep the weight above your head for the entire set, alternating arms each set
- **Tempo**: slow
- **Repetitions:** 10

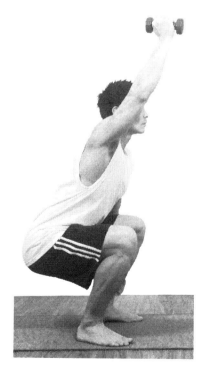

Figure 52: Single Arm Overhead Squat

Swiss Ball Squat

- Place a Swiss ball between your lower back and a wall
- Take a comfortable stance, arms at your sides. Keep your feet shoulder width apart and slightly turned out so that your knees align with the second toe
- Inhale and then lower yourself down into a squat as you breathe out. Go as low as you comfortably can, then inhale as you return to standing
- Breathe through your nose if you can. If you need to breathe out through your mouth, purse your lips to keep a little tension in them
- **Tempo**: slow
- **Repetitions:** 10

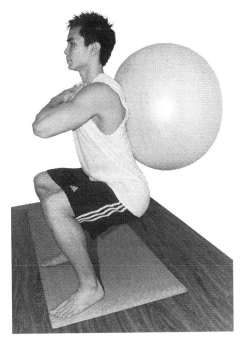

Figure 53: Ball Squat

Quadratus Lumborum Stabilization

Quadratus Lumborum is an important stabilizer of the lower spine.

- Begin in side-lying position
- Prop up on your elbow and then lift the pelvis off the mat, supporting the lower body with the side of the knee nearest to the mat (Fig. 54-A)
- Maintain this position as long as possible (for a minimum of 20 sec)
- Advance to supporting the upper body with the hand (straight arm) and side of the foot on the mat (Fig. 54-B)

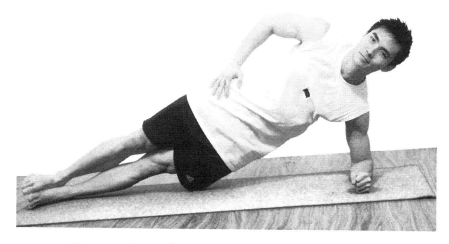

Figure 54: Quadratus Lumborum Stabilization

Swiss Ball Side Flexion

Side bending exercises are also used if there is a scoliosis. When there is a lumbar curve, the muscles on the convex side are usually stretched and weakened. Therefore lying on a Swiss ball on the concave side will help to strengthen the weak muscles on the convex side. If unsure, then test each side of the body and then concentrate on the weaker side.

- Sit on a Swiss ball with your feet at the junction of a wall and the floor
- Slowly rotate over the ball so one of your hips is squarely on top of the ball and your feet are securely anchored against the wall; the upper thigh of the top leg should be in line with your body
- While lying sideways over the ball with your arms at your sides, slowly raise yourself sideways until your body is perpendicular to the floor; reverse the motion until you are once again at the starting position. Visualize curling up sideways one vertebra at a time, starting with your head

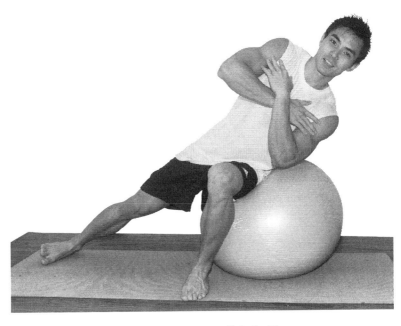

Figure 55: Swiss Ball Side Flexion

Wall Push Up

- Stand about two feet away from a wall
- Place your hands on the wall about chest width apart at shoulder level
- Draw your navel in, keep your body straight and drop your weight towards the wall
- Push into the wall to return to the starting position again keeping your body in perfect alignment
- When you can perform more than 20 repetitions with perfect form, move your feet farther away from the wall

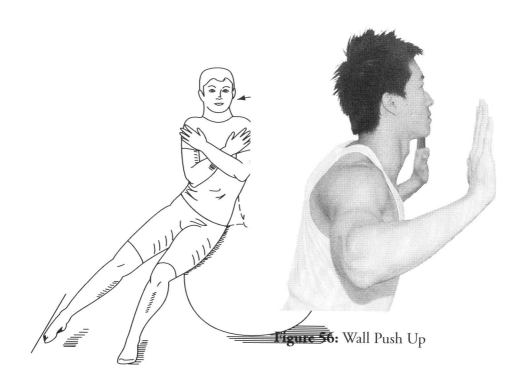

Figure 56: Wall Push Up

Seated Bend Pull

- Sit on a swiss ball and hold a cable or elastic cord out in front of you
- Breathe out and bend forward, keeping a natural curve in your lower back; do not let your back round as you bend forward
- As you inhale, return to the starting position and bring your arms up toward your chest in a rowing motion. Do not shrug your shoulders

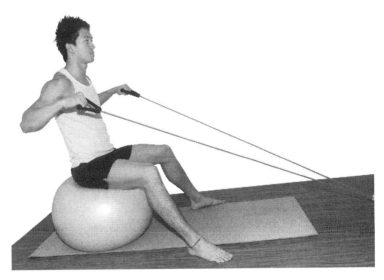

Figure 57: Seated Bend Pull

How to Build Your Own Scoliosis Exercise Program

Your exercise program for scoliosis can be as flexible as you want. The primary goal must be to improve your health and restore some balance back into your spine and muscles.

It has been observed that in some male patients, scoliosis regresses spontaneously. Since this phenomenon is observed more often in males than in female patients, one reason for this could be the greater opportunities for physical exercise that exist for males more than females in our society. Therefore some exercise is always better than none.

Undoubtedly, the program needs to be tailored to your age, health, and need profile, obviously an area where your chiropractor or physical therapist can help and guide you best. However, the basic requirement of a versatile program is that you must be able to do it on a regular basis either two to three times a week for optimal results.

Selecting the Right Exercise Plan

We have already discussed this section exhaustively. Flip to the reader's resource section given at the end of this book for more help.

Begin by mapping out your tight areas with the help of the diagram given in Chapter 12 (Fig. 13). Your chiropractor can recommend adjustments to your basic program based on the two commonly seen curves: the S or the C-shaped scoliosis. After six to eight weeks of exercising and dietary changes, reassess the progress made and if everything is going according to plan, you can continue to the next level. Regardless of whether you have an S or a C-shaped scoliosis, the exercises outlined in this book can be done by anyone. However, do flip through Chapter 15 again for an action plan that will guide you into building your own safe diet and exercise program.

Ease Into It

The biggest mistake many of us make when getting back to exercise is overdoing it… or what i call the guilt response. When we get off track, our first response is often to jump back in and do twice as much work to make up for what we missed. But there are a number of problems with that response:

Loss of Strength and Endurance

If you've been off exercise for more than a month, you've lost some of that strength and endurance you once had. As a result, your body won't be capable of doing the same level of training you were doing before.

Injuries and Delayed Onset Muscle Soreness

Going full-speed with your workouts from the start means you'll be experiencing plenty of muscle soreness, and if you keep trying to work out when you're very sore, you run the risk of injuring yourself.

Dreading Your Workouts

If you do too much too soon and you're sore, tired and fatigued, you may start to dread your workouts and that's not the attitude you want when trying to get back on track.

CHAPTER 17

Living with Scoliosis

"Motivation is what gets you started. Habit is what keeps you going."

— *Jim Ryun*

Caring For Your Back

More than 50 percent of all Americans will suffer from some sort of back problem at some time during their lives. Some problems may be congenital, such as scoliosis, while others may be the result of a car accident, fall or sporting injury (in which case the pain may subside, only to reappear years later). Most back problems are due to tension and muscular tightness, which come from poor posture, being overweight, inactivity and lack of core stability.

Stretching and abdominal exercises can help your back if done with common sense. If you have a back problem, consult a reliable physician who will test to see exactly where the problem lies. Ask your physician which of the stretches and exercises shown in this book would be most help to you.

Anyone with a history of lower back problem should avoid stretches called hyperextensions that arch the back. They create too much stress on the lower back.

The British Chiropractic Association states that 32% of people spend 10 hours or more a day in a seated position, and that half of these people do not ever leave their desks, not even for lunch. Many people sit once they go home from work as well, further contributing to lower back strain.

The best way to take care of your back is to use proper methods of stretching, strengthening, standing and sitting. It is what you do day to day that determines your health. In the following pages are some suggestions for back care.

Lifting

Never lift anything (heavy or light) with your legs straight, bending only your back. Always bend your knees so the bulk of the work is done by the big muscles of your legs and not the small muscles of your lower back. Keep the weight close to your body and your back as straight as possible.

Sitting

For the last century, work chairs in schools, factories and offices have been designed for sitting upright, with the hip, knees and ankles all at right angles. Until recently, it was widely believed that people sat with a 90-degree bending of the hip joints while preserving lordosis (concavity) of the back. This has since been proven untrue.

New research carried out by Scottish and Canadian researchers shows that sitting with your back at a 90 degree angle to your hips places strain on your vertebrae and contributes to back pain. The research, carried out in Scotland, examined 22 healthy volunteers using a positional MRI machine. The positional MRI machine differs from a traditional MRI in that patients can assume positions other than lying on their back. Having the patients assume different positions allowed the researchers to determine at what angle spinal disc movement was greatest. Disc movement was found to be greatest when the spine was at a 90 degree angle (i.e. the volunteer was sitting upright). Disc movement was least when the volunteers leaned back in their chairs so that their spine was at a 135 degree angle. The researchers concluded that sitting with your back at a 135 degree angle is best for back health. Because this angle is difficult to maintain without sliding forward on the chair, Dr. Bashir of the University of Alberta Hospital in Canada, who headed the study, stated that an angle of 120 degrees or less may be more practical.

Seating Positions

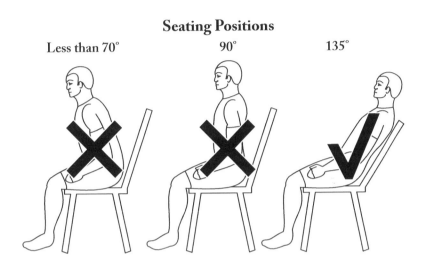

Figure 58: Correct sitting postures

Standing

Do not stand with your knees locked into a straight position. This tilts your pelvis forward and puts the pressure of standing directly on your lower back, a position of weakness. Let your leg muscles control your posture when standing by having the knees slightly bent and feet pointed straight ahead.

Prevention Key to a Healthy Spine

The greatest tip I can offer to anyone suffering from back pain is to not ignore it! Pain is necessary to prevent further damage to joints and alerts us that something is not right. As in most cases, prevention is the key to maintaining a healthy spine as you head into your older years. Timing is critical in muscle, ligament, and joint injury because healing begins immediately after the damage. If activity is not started soon, usually between two and six weeks, then injured tissues may not recover their flexibility, strength, and ability to function (i.e., to do what they are designed to do). After losing flexibility and function, the healed tissues become weak. Even small movements can then lead to re-injury and to a chronic back problem and, eventually, to degeneration. Just as your teeth need to be brushed daily to keep them in top notch condition, your spine also requires maintenance. A large number of spinal problems I see in practice could have been prevented with proper treatment immediately after the initial injury.

Protect yourself from strain and disability by following these simple tips.

1. **Listen to Your Back**

   Pain is a warning sign. Your body is telling you that you have already or are about to cause damage. If what you are doing hurts, then STOP. Do not try to push through the pain.

2. **Exercise**

   Regular exercise is important to help maintain mobility and strength. It should be done without pain and it should be done regularly. Brisk walking, swimming and cycling are all excellent exercises, but you should do what is suitable for you and what you enjoy. You are more apt to exercise if you enjoy the activity you are participating in.

3. **Warm Up**

   You should warm up your body before any form of physical activity, whether it is nursing, sports or gardening. This prepares the body for action and helps to prevent injuries.

4. **Cool Down**

   Cooling down and stretching after exercise or physical activity is just as important as a warm up. Never "bounce" your stretches and do it gently without pain.

5. **Move Now And Then**

   Whether you are at home, at work or in the car, prolonged sitting causes pressure on the discs and weakness of the muscles. Get up and move every now and then, even if it is only for a minute. The body is designed for movement, not for slouching in front of the TV or driving for hours on end.

6. **Sleep Properly**

   Sleep in a comfortable position. On your side in the "foetal" position is usually the least stressful on your back. Too many people with scoliosis worry about which side of the curve they should be lying on to prevent aggravating their condition. Lying on either side in the "foetal" position rarely affects your curve, yet not getting a good night's rest will definitely affect your health and spine. More caution should be reserved for sleeping on your front as it puts the most stress on your back and neck and can lead to trouble. Using a pillow of the right height which supports the neck is also important.

7. **Use Medication Wisely**

   All drugs have side effects so they should be used wisely and conservatively. The use of pain killers (paracetamol, Co-codamol etc.) and non steroidal anti-inflammatory drugs (nurofen, brufen, diclofenac etc.) only helps to mask the symptoms and do not address the cause of the problem. Use them as sparingly as possible and never over a long period of time.

8. **Consult Your Chiropractor or Spinal Professional**

   If you have a long term problem, whether it is just an annoyance or disabling, or if you have a recurring problem, then chiropractic treatment can probably help. Chiropractors can usually give you marked relief from pain and discomfort and improved quality of life, as well as decreasing the likelihood of a recurrence. Try to find a chiropractor which is familiar with treating scoliosis.

Don't Let Pain Hold You Back

Constant pain can be wearing, both physically and mentally. Two common responses to pain can make a bad situation even worse:

The first is trying to ignore your pain by attempting to mask it with drugs. Particularly since it became known that COX-2 inhibitors (Vioxx, Bextra, Celebrex) have been taken off the market because they can contribute to a higher risk of heart attack, many people who suffer chronic pain have had to turn to the use of narcotic analgesics to manage their pain. These drugs, such as Oxycontin, Morphine and Oxycodone, are highly addictive and can cause many problems of their own such as constipation, sleepiness, and inability to perform normal activities of life.

The second is to limit activities so as not to aggravate the pain. Unfortunately, limiting activities also limits your enjoyment of life and can be very maladaptive over time. People who choose this route choose to allow their pain to dictate how they live their lives, often gradually withdrawing from all activities which aggravate their pain.

When you limit yourself in this way, either by using harmful drugs or severely limiting your lifestyle, you are robbing yourself of any ability to enjoy your life. You are cheating yourself of good health as well, because eventually this unhealthy lifestyle will begin to affect other aspects of your health. For example, if you are unable to exercise you may gain weight, putting your heart at risk.

Truly, your only option is to act on the cause, or root, of your pain. Although this may seem a Herculean task, it is your best and only option to preserve your health and gain some enjoyment from your life. However, this is a decision that you must make on your own. Live with your pain, or embrace life — the choice is yours.

Getting Rid Of Muscular Pain

Have you heard of *trigger points* (TrPs)?

Research by Drs. Janet Travell and David Simons, authors of "The Trigger Point Manual" reveals that trigger points are the primary cause of pain in at least 75% of pain conditions, which, if I may add, also includes pain caused by scoliosis.

Trigger points are, in effect, a kind of muscle stiffness that may cause tiny contraction knots to develop in the surrounding muscle and tissue, whenever a portion of the body is injured or overworked. These should not be ignored because trigger points typically issue their pain to some other place in the body, which is why conventional treatments for pain so often fail. This brings us to the next query...

What Triggers Trigger Points?

Trigger points can occur as a result of muscle trauma (from car accidents, falls, sports- and work-related injuries, etc.), muscle strain from repetitive movements at work or play, postural strain from standing or sitting improperly for long periods at the computer, emotional stress, anxiety, allergies, nutritional deficiencies, inflammation, and toxins in the environment. A single event can create a trigger point, and you can suffer the effects of the event the rest of your life if that trigger point is not addressed and addressed quickly.

How Can You Tell if You Have Trigger Points?

If you feel lingering, nagging pain, tightness, or restriction in any part of your body, the indication is that those are the effects of a trigger point. Trigger points may produce symptoms as diverse as dizziness, earaches, sinusitis, nausea, heartburn, false heart pain, heart arrhythmia, genital pain, and numbness in the hands and feet.

Travell and Simons argue in their book, and I am convinced by their logic, that trigger points can bring on headaches, neck and jaw pain, lower back pain, sciatica, tennis elbow, and carpal tunnel syndrome. Trigger points could also be the source of joint pain in the shoulder, wrist, hip, knee, and ankle that is often mistaken for arthritis, tendinitis, bursitis, or ligament injury. All this is well documented in "Why We Hurt: A Complete Physical & Spiritual Guide to Healing Your Chronic Pain" by Dr. Greg Fors, in which he explains precisely why so many different conditions are rooted in trigger points.

How to Address Your Trigger Points

The solution lies in Trigger Point Therapy that you can learn to apply on yourself, or you may seek the help of a trained therapist.

The therapy, which is a form of massage, will immediately result in soft tissue release, allowing for increased blood flow, a reduction in muscle spasm, and the break-up of your scar tissues. In the process, it will also eliminate any build-up of toxic metabolic waste from your blood stream. In this fashion, your body will undergo a neurological release, a marked reduction in the pain signals to the brain and a resetting of your neuromuscular system for maximum relief.

Remember that your spine and muscles surrounding the spine is one of the most important part of your body. If you injure your spine, get back into light physical activity whilst making sure not to aggravate the pain. Stay physically active to keep your spine moving so that it stays nourished and hydrated. This will speed up your recovery process.

Mapping Out Your Trigger Points

Myofascial trigger points are extremely sore points that can occur in taut ropy bands throughout the body. They may feel like painful lumps or nodules, and they restrict range of motion. Because they are found in so many places in the body, tight myofascia can cause a vast array of symptoms. Single trigger points (TrP) can occur in anyone. If there are one or more TrPs perpetuating factors, the TrPs may seem to spread. TrP perpetuating factors include anything that will continually lead to stress on the muscle, including trauma, body asymmetry, or co-existing conditions.

When you have a trigger point in a muscle, it causes pain at the end of range of motion when you stretch that muscle, and it weakens the muscle even before it causes pain. Your ankle, knee or hip may buckle, or your grip may fail, depending on which muscle is involved (these symptoms are *not* part of Fibromyalgia.) You then avoid stretching this muscle because it hurts. Muscles are designed to work best with motion. When you don't stretch the muscle, it becomes less healthy and your range of motion decreases. Circulation in your capillaries, your *microcirculation*, becomes impaired around the TrP. Nutrients and oxygen can't be delivered easily, nor wastes removed. Your lymph system depends on muscle movement to move toxins out of the body, so that system begins to stagnate as well. Other muscles do the work of the TrP-weakened muscle.

Self Treatment of Trigger Points

1. Locate your trigger points so you know where to massage. Usually, you're able to feel a trigger point just by moving your fingers along a muscle until you feel an especially taut area. Keep moving along this tightness until you find the spot that's especially tender to your touch. If you move over a recently developed trigger point, the muscle twitches, but chronic trigger points just feel tight. Using the body diagram in Figure 59, mark the trigger points you find.

2. Focus on a single pressure point at a time when you do your self-massage. This helps relieve the stress on related trigger points, making them easier to treat.

3. Feel your muscle to determine the direction of the fibers. If you can determine the direction, stroke the muscle in that direction with your fingertips or thumbs. Use short strokes down the entire length of the muscle, covering it just once. If you can't determine the direction, move to the next step.

4. Zero in on the trigger pain with a kneading, circular massage stroke. Use enough pressure that you experience mild discomfort in the muscle, but not so much that you experience real pain.

5. Leave the pressure point alone after you massage it with about twelve kneading strokes. Return to it later in the day, using the same massage process. Trigger points respond better to frequent treatment than they do to extended treatment.

6. Move on to the next trigger point if you have multiple areas that you want to treat with massage.

As a rule of thumb, remember to only attempt the low-impact exercises for curves greater than 20 degrees. High-impact exercises such as light jogs or tennis can be done occasionally for curves less than 20 degrees, but only if you don't experience any pain. If you do, discontinue immediately.

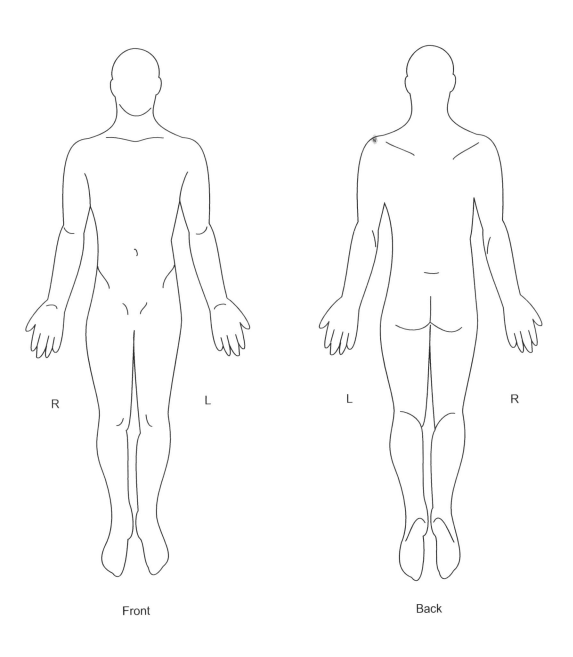

R   L   L   R

Front   Back

Figure 59: Mark out your trigger points (✖)

Exercises to Avoid While Going Through Correction

High-impact exercise requires both feet to be lifted off the ground simultaneously. Some examples would include running, jumping, and jump rope. High-impact activities do strengthen the bones and develop more endurance, power, agility and coordination than low-impact activities, but reserve these for later in the program once the curve has improved below 20 degrees, and after you have fallen into a routine with an exercise program.

While doing the exercises mentioned above, if the deformity becomes visually worse (such as increasing the curve, pelvic or shoulder imbalance), then these exercises should be avoided. Make sure a mirror is present so that you can monitor yourself closely or get a partner to watch.

In general, remember to:

Avoid any kind of back-bending exercises such as the "Prone Cobra" pose done in yoga. These may cause severe strain on your curved spine and may worsen the problem.

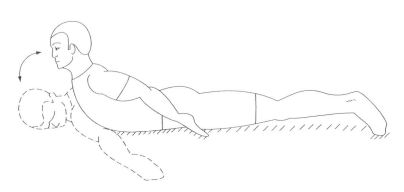

Figure 60: Prone Cobra - Exercise to avoid

Low Impact Exercises for Scoliosis

These are ideally suitable for:

- People with injuries in the joints, bones or connective tissue such as scoliosis
- Pregnant women
- Chronic sufferers of problems like arthritis, osteoporosis or stress fractures
- Obese patients
- Those who have a strong aversion to high impact exercises
- General spinal maintenance after correction

In addition to the exercises described in this book, the following are just a few of the most popular low impact activities which you can add to your regular exercise routine.

Swimming in Fresh Water

Swimming is highly recommended to scoliosis sufferers of all ages. Apart from being a beneficial exercise, it also promotes increased lung function, which can be impeded by curvature of the spine. If you decide on being treated by bracing, the freedom of swimming has an added psychological benefit, after being contained inside a rigid jacket for hours each day.

Swimming is one of the best exercises on the planet, working all the major muscles, but it poses the challenge of exposing you to the large amounts of chlorine that are in most swimming pools. However, you still have the option of swimming in fresh waters or ocean depending on the temperature of the water.

Brisk Walking

Here are a few tips on how to get the most out of your walking routine:

Make It Brisk

Walking briskly assists in increasing your heart rate, helping you to maximize your cardiovascular potential and burn calories.

Try Interval Training

By adding short bursts of speed or an occasional steep hill to your walking workouts, you can increase the intensity of your workouts as well as your calorie-burn. Try hill climbing workouts on the treadmill, or one of the beginner interval workouts to get started.

Use Your Arms

Make sure you're not holding onto the treadmill, and when you're outside, swing your arms to keep the intensity up. Holding weights as you walk is a no-no (it can cause injury), but consider using walking poles as a safe alternative.

Mix Things Up

If walking is your sole source of cardio, cross-train with other activities to keep challenging your body.

Walking Up the Stairs

Believe it or not, walking up the stairs can be an incredibly intense workout. If you're a beginner, try adding a few minutes of stair climbing to your usual workout, or hop on the step mill at the gym for a quick five minutes towards the end of your workout.

Adding Intensity to Your Workouts

Once you are settled into a daily routine of low-impact exercises, it's time for you to graduate to the next level. Try some of these ideas for making your low-impact exercises more intense:

Add Upper Body Movements.

Choose aerobics or gym machines with upper body options like a cross-country ski machine or elliptical trainer.

Go Faster

Try to pick up the pace, whether you're walking, cycling or paragliding.

Make Elaborate Movements

Another way to add intensity is to vigorously swing your arms from side to side while walking; or abruptly you could break into a dancing gig, particularly if you have a walkman to your ear.

Don't Forget to Involve Your Lower Body

Add walking lunges or side steps with squats to your usual walking routine.

Exercise Equipment

Three pieces of equipment that I have found useful for my patients who have scoliosis are a vibration machine, an inversion table, and a portable traction device called a Dynamic Brace System. All are good in introducing forces into your spine to either help by stimulating new bone formation or unloading the spinal discs. While the inversion table is in no way nearly as effective as the Dynamic Brace System I utilize in practice, the benefits lie in the fact that they are readily found in sporting stores and can be used at home. Here is a brief explanation of these types of equipment.

Inversion Table If you have a curvature of less than 20 degrees, an inversion table is an affordable piece of equipment that you could invest in. While it may not offer correction for curves that are higher than 20 degrees, it may help to prevent worsening of the scoliosis due to gravity and daily wear and tear. Some of the benefits are as follows:

- **Maintains your height** — Regularly inverting will help you avoid the "shrinkage" that naturally occurs as a result of gravity over a lifetime.
- **Improves circulation** — When you're inverted, your blood circulation is aided by gravity rather than having to work against it. Additionally, with inversion, gravity helps the lymphatic system clear faster, easing the aches and pains of stiff muscles.
- **Relieves stress** — An inversion table provides the same feeling of relaxation as a yoga class - with a lot less effort.
- **Heightens mental alertness** — Any upside-down activity increases the supply of oxygen to the brain, which many experts believe helps maintain mental sharpness.
- **Increases flexibility and range of motion** — With inversion, your joints stay healthy and supple, meaning you can remain as active as you were in your younger years.
- **Improves posture** — The stretching that comes with reversing the force of gravity on your body helps you sit, stand, and move with more ease and grace.
- **Realigns the spine after workouts** — During inversion, minor misalignments often correct themselves naturally, which is not possible with running or other aerobic exercises.

Here are five innovative ways of using your Inversion Table:

1. **Inverted Squats** — In the full inverted position, you can use your buttock muscles (glutes) and hamstrings to pull yourself up; the motion would be simply trying to bend your legs at your knees.

2. **Inverted Crunch** — In the full inverted position, place your hands on your chest and use your abs to lift your upper body about one-third of the way up.

3. **Inverted sit-up** — In the full inverted position, extend your arms as if you were reaching for your feet and try to touch your feet; some experts say that one inverted sit-up is equivalent to 10 regular sit-ups.

4. **Increase the decompression** — In the full inverted position, grab the table legs and pull down; this way you can increase and control the amount of decompression if you want or need more. This is particularly good for people with scoliosis.

5. **Inverted Rotation** — In the full inverted position, reach with the opposite hand for the table legs and pull yourself into rotation; you can then switch hands and do the same for the opposite side.

Vibration Machine

I read somewhere that the first studies on vibration equipment were done on military personnel and Russian Olympic athletes. They used a special mechanical vibrating plate adjusted to the right frequency so that when people stood on it, it caused the postural muscles to contract anywhere from 30 to 50 times a second.

As the body ever so slightly shifts back and forth, the muscles must contract and relax with each shift. So, in just 10 minutes, three times a week of standing on the plate, your muscles build up greater strength, stability, and tone.

You could use it in two ways. You can either do it separately or, as I do, stand on the vibrator and let it work for you, while you busy yourself with other weight-bearing exercises — such as lunges, leg lifts, and pushups. These exercises will gently pull on the tendons that connect your muscles to your bones, while stimulating your osteoblasts, which are your "bone builders."

There is research that suggests that when you exercise on a vibrating surface, it helps increase muscle strength 20-30 percent more than conventional strength training. I've received a lot of positive feedback from my patients who use this machine in my practice, and I use it in conjunction with the Dynamic Brace System to correct curvatures greater than 20 degrees.

Dynamic Brace System

The Dynamic Brace System known as D.B.S., is a dynamic portable traction like corset that fits around your back. It works by applying three-dimensional traction and allows for vertical and horizontal traction as well as symmetrical and asymmetrical traction. It was developed to aid the sufferers of herniated discs and low back and sciatic pain, however, because of the three-dimensional traction, this means that it can correct a swayed back or a flat back in addition to scoliosis.

I highly recommend this device to patients who suffer from progressive scoliosis such as an adolescent who has not reached skeletal maturity or anyone with a curvature that is more than 20 degrees. The great news is the D.B.S. is effective on correcting scoliosis as well as preventing further curvature of the spine because it has a horizontal pressure force which can be moved and adjust the horizontal pressure pad according to the patient's condition.

The D.B.S. is so easy to use that patients requiring long-term care may easily be taught by a trained health care practitioner how to administer self-treatments at home. Treatments thus become more convenient and patients feel that they have more control over their lives. Be sure to get an X-ray before you begin using the D.B.S. and 6 months after to record any changes that have occurred in your spine.

Clinical studies have proven that the D.B.S. can improve your range of motion, lessen your back pain, and correct the curvature of the spine. I have personally seen great results in my patients and often use the D.B.S. in conjunction with diet changes and exercise.

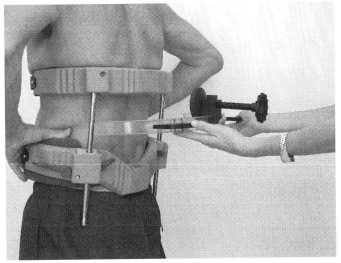

Figure 61: Vertebtrac with Dynamic Brace System

Recommend Usage:

In patients with a curve greater than 20 degrees, when the scoliosis is progressive, it's recommended that you perform daily treatments of 30 minutes with D.B.S. until maturity of the spine is reached. The traction power applied should be between 10-20kg. on each side. This, of course, can vary according to the age and the constitution of each patient.

For patients who have no pain or other complaints but have a tendency for progression such as adolescents, it's recommended that you treat your scoliosis with the D.B.S. for 30 minutes, 1 or 2 times daily until skeletal maturity is reached and the person's curvature remains stable for 2 - 3 years.

In patients with curvatures greater than 30 degrees or suffer from pain, the D.B.S. treatment is started immediately for 30 minutes, 3 times per day. Once skeletal maturity is reached, 1 or 2 30-minute treatments should be continued daily for a period of six months. X-rays should be taken every 6 months with a healthcare professional to document the changes in the curve. If you discover a scoliosis progression greater than 5 degrees then this requires a resumption of 30-minute treatments, 3 times a daily until progression is halted and the scoliosis is stable, which is confirmed with a spinal X-ray.

Remember, however, that while the Dynamic Brace System has been proven to be beneficial, it is best to start slow, as with any other exercise explained in this book, while gradually building your momentum for more vigorous exercises later. Plunging headlong into any high-impact exercise will make your body feel more sore than relaxed. So please resist the temptation to go full throttle into any exercise routine that you eventually choose for yourself.

Testimonial: D.B.S. for Scoliosis Correction

"I have been using the Dynamic Bracing System for one year with alarming results. Cases ranging from 44-degree scoliosis to the most severe disc ruptures all resulting in dramatic symptomatic and physiological changes. How did I do it? I combined the Vertetrac with specific isolated exercises, specific stretching, massage, trigger point ultrasound, and forced manipulation. When they are all combined in one visit, then the results are shocking, usually within six months or less. If you are interested in treating the most severe cases with phenomenal results, then do your research and purchase a Vertetrac brace today."

— *Dr Louis Salvagio, DC, CCRD, PT*
Associate Professor, University of St. Augustine

Remember to be patient and consistent. Exert caution; don't expect overnight changes and your body will begin to respond in time.

However, for that to happen, you must first learn to take responsibility for your health. Don't leave everything to your health professional. Seek professional help by all means, but more than the professionals, you need to understand the demands of your body and how it works. Only then will you be able to help your scoliosis.

Believe me, our bodies are incredible machines. If you maintain and oil them properly, they will last longer, function more efficiently and won't suffer from the wear and tear of aging.

Tips on how to incorporate exercise into your lifestyle

It's indeed very simple. To begin with, choose an exercise plan that:

1. **You enjoy**
2. **Is fun to do**
3. **Is affordable**
4. **Suits your particular lifestyle**

For instance, if time is a constraint, choose something like a half-hour of brisk walking every day, cycling from home, or swimming on the way back from school or work. If you can, make it a family activity, so you can have more fun.

When something becomes a part of your lifestyle, habit drives you regardless of how you are feeling that day, just like brushing your teeth or taking a bath. Exercising is the same principle. Here are some more ways to add exercise into your daily routine:

- Take the stairs instead of lifts or elevators
- If you work in a large office, walk to talk to your colleagues, rather than picking up the phone

- If you use buses, get off a stop or two earlier and walk
- Don't worry if you are unable to park next to the supermarket or shop entrance. Further down the road will be less crowded!
- For small amounts of shopping or other errands use a bicycle instead of the car; this will save you money and the hassle of finding a place to park
- If you have a cordless phone, walk and talk
- For every outdoor activity, find one indoor activity for bad weather days

Bide Your Time

Decide how often you are going to exercise in a week, choose the most convenient days and times of day and set aside those times as sacrosanct.

Be Consistent

You need at least 30 minutes of exercise a day to experience any weight loss benefits. Major studies have shown that 60 minutes a day is actually best. Ideally, the exercise should be continuous, but it could be split up into two 30-minute intervals.

Build Up Your Momentum Gradually

Don't try and do too much too soon, otherwise you may feel unwell and lose motivation to continue. The key to successful exercising is to start slowly, particularly if you have led a sedentary lifestyle. You will finish your exercise with a sense of achievement, feel better and give yourself the motivation to continue. It is also essential to start slowly in order to prevent injury.

Keep a Diary

Keeping a diary of your exercise (i.e. how much time, how often and how difficult) can keep you motivated as you see your progress. A diary can also be useful in deciding when to increase your exercise in terms of frequency, time and intensity.

Invest in Good Equipment

If you choose to walk, it is very important to invest in a good pair of walking shoes which offer support for your spine, hips, knees, ankles and feet. If you progress to jogging, it is even more essential that you invest in a pair of good running shoes.

Set Clear Goals

Set yourself short-term goals and be realistic. For example, you may aim to increase the time you walk from 10 minutes to 15 minutes. You set your threshold and then go about increasing it gradually.

Exercise in Company

It helps to exercise with a partner or a friend, whose company you enjoy. It will keep you both motivated and checking on each other's progress.

Wear Appropriate Clothes

Wear comfortable clothes which helps your skin breathe through the pores.

Try Music Therapy

Carry a portable music player and listen to your favorite music or audiobooks, as you exercise.

Above All, Listen to Your Body

If exercise worsens symptoms, modify your program, or if need be, stop. As your energy and health improve, you will be able to tolerate larger amounts of the aerobic exercise, which will lead to weight loss.

A good chiropractor or physical therapist who is familiar with treating scoliosis can guide you through the specifics of a good exercise program. If you do use a personal trainer, please be aware that many don't understand the nutritional principles, so it would be wise to double-check his/her recommendations with your chiropractor.

Last But Not the Least… Stick With the Plan!

No one can motivate you, if you yourself are not willing. Rather than having an all-or-nothing attitude towards exercise, think of it as an ongoing process. There may be days when you have to unavoidably miss your exercise such as when you are ill. It doesn't matter. Just continue when you can.

Remember: Whatever you do, don't exercise until two or three hours after a meal. It is important to drink water before, during and after exercise to keep your body hydrated. Don't exercise strenuously during very hot or humid weather.

During exercise, if you feel sore or ache, rest if you feel the need to. If the pain persists, check with your healthcare professional.

Personal Story: Growing Up with Scoliosis

"In year six, the government sent nurses to each school to do a health check up on all the students. But I was the only one being called out to a tiny room. The nurses inside all looked at me with a worried look. I never forget that day. They asked me to bend down and confirmed that I have scoliosis. I was sent to the General Hospital and was told by the doctor to wear a brace to stabilize the condition.

"Initially wearing the brace was very painful. The hard plastic edge of the brace was always cutting my flesh, especially on both sides of the hip bones. It hurt so much even when I move my body, let alone walking. Over time, the flesh gave way, the skin there becomes loose and disfigured from the rubbing of the brace. As I have to wear the brace almost 23 hours every day, the skin trapped inside the brace became different and tore off easily. The sweat trapped inside the brace worsens it all. The smell of it was horrid and I can still remember till now. I always felt so hot and itchy when I started to sweat. But once I scratched it, I regretted it so badly. For the braced skin had deteriorated and became so fragile and weak that once being scratch, it tears off so easily. And the wound could even ooze out yellowish discharge and sometimes even blood. It made the smell even horrid. I felt like one walking corpse. The doctor could do nothing. Even I myself despised my own body. But I could not go without the brace. I still have to force myself to wear it. It was the only hope I had during that time to escape from operation.

"In secondary school, my personality had changed. I became quiet, always hiding in the shadows. Everyone, including the teachers would give me a look. It was the weird look of pity they gave me that made me feel I was a freak. Being isolated, I soon become the easy target of school bullies. I was only a freak in their eyes. I went through all this at the age of 13, alone and quietly. The most painful part of wearing the brace is not my body, but my heart.

"When I was 19, the doctor discharged me. He said my condition had stabilized and can go without the brace. It was the happiest day of my life. Thereafter, my skin recovered fully and is now all velvet smooth. But the backache that I suffered while I was on brace continues to torment me. I tried massages, heat therapy, and plasters, but they only provided temporary relief. When I was 24, I went back to my doctor whom set up his own clinic in Mount Elizabeth Hospital. But he said I have scoliosis, it cannot be helped. I can only live with the severe backache.

"In 2009, God asked me to get up from bed one night to check my e-mail. I did not understand as I rarely check my e-mail. But I obey. And I saw Dr. Kevin Lau website. It openned up my eyes and I thought it is too good too wonderful to be true. Doubts and fear set in. For all these years I was used to live in hopelessness. And all of a sudden, hope appears out of nowhere. It is the of taking that step forward to hold on to that hope. Everyone around me is skeptical about it. After months, I finally took up the courage to call Dr Lau's Clinic.

"On the first visit, Dr Kevin is kind, humble and caring. But it is the confidence in him that he can correct my scoliosis that makes me believe in miracle. To me, he is an inspiration himself. Without further ado, I took up a program for correction. I was totally committed. He taught me that exercise and nutrition play an important role too. He could lend me books to educate me on my own self healing. He is always so willing to teach me whatever I asked. He would diligently put up articles on his website and health blog to educate his patients for our own health being. He was being interviewed on radio, on TV and on newspapers. His book contains all the knowledge we scoliosis sufferers need to know comprehensively. It also contained evolutionary truths that will improve our health greatly.

"During the treatments, my posture improved greatly and I do not slouch anymore. I followed his recommended diet, and I experience great change. My eyesight improved from 500 to 450 degrees over the 6 month period. My stamina improved greatly and I do not get so tired and restless easily. I do not fall sick, which I usually do. My skin complexion improve so much that I need no makeup anymore. Everyone find me getting taller too. My backache also improved over time. Most importantly, I gained back my self confidence.

"After six months treatments, my upper curve of my 'S' shaped spine improved from 36 to 30 degrees. The lower curve improved from 35 to 26 degrees. The total 15 degrees is a miracle to me. It is a dream comes true. My hope was fulfilled. I am deeply in great multitude of gratitude to Dr Kevin.

"Not only correcting my scoliosis, he imparted his relentlessly strong positive belief that changed my whole outlook in life. All things are possible if you dare to believe."

— *Colleen M. (29 years old)*

CHAPTER 18

Putting It All Together - How to Use This Book

"The secret to getting ahead is getting started."

— *Mark Twain*

C oming to the end of my labor of love, I know that there is a lot to take in.

I also know that you are eager to start correcting your scoliosis, right away. However, please refrain from jumping straight into the exercise portion of this book, without first assimilating and understanding the nutritional aspect.

The insight gained from the nutrition section of this book will address the biochemical imbalance that is contributing to your scoliosis; while the exercises and stretches will help with structural imbalances that are already present in your spine. The two of them together, diet and exercise, are a "dynamic duo" that carry great strength in partnership rather than individually.

Further, don't feel the need to make all the changes that I have suggested in this book overnight. Your scoliosis didn't happen overnight, so the healing process won't come about overnight. Rome was built brick by brick while your spine will also be built back, cell by cell.

Expect changes to come slowly initially. Don't rush into this program. Stick to your diet and exercise plan for the long term, rather than jumping in hard and fast. Take it from me that when you gradually switch to healthier foods, your taste buds will mature and begin to appreciate and enjoy the wholesome foods over sugary, fried stuff from the past. From my years of experience with my patients, most turn out to be very picky eaters, but after following my program they have come to prefer whole foods over comfort or junk foods. But it takes time.

Finding a naturopath or nutritionist familiar with Metabolic Typing® will help you make   this transition smoothly. The good news is that the more positive changes you make with regard to your eating and exercise habits, the better you will feel, and the more energy you will have at your disposal to happily course through the rest of your journey from scoliosis to health.

After performing the previously described procedure for locating and diagramming your curve and the associated areas of muscle tightness and pain, I encourage you to take this book to a chiropractor, osteopath or back care therapist who is familiar with scoliosis and discuss in detail an appropriate exercise program for your scoliosis type.

By all means, ask your back care professional for guidance before you begin exercising. If you have severe osteoporosis, nerve or joint pain, be sure to consult your therapist before beginning this or any other program.

Over the following few pages, I have broken down the book into a more manageable action plan for beginners and advance level readers.

Beginners can start by building the proper foundations for a healthy diet and exercise regime right away. Try following the suggestions outlined over one to three months (or maybe more) at your own pace before moving on to the advanced section. Remain alert to your body's whispers. It may be trying to tell you something. Stay alert to all the changes that you notice in your body and adjust or tweak your plan accordingly.

Once you are familiar with the suggestions in the beginner's action plan, it's now time to fine tuning your body's demands for optimal health in the advanced action plan. By this stage, you should have a regular exercise routine and a rough idea of what foods are good and which are bad for you. This section of the program will require you to get to know how your body works. You might even be surprised at its amazing ability to adapt and heal as you continue to strive for optimal health.

Beginner's Nutritional Plan

☐ First and foremost, complete the step-by-step instructions on Scoliosis Home Screen on page 38 to find out if you have scoliosis. Complete the questions and then draw out what you find on page 40 (Fig. 4).

☐ Begin to gradually eliminate all processed foods and metabolic disruptors listed in the Table 4 on page 327, even before learning your Metabolic Type®

☐ Avoid processed foods, sugar, refined flour and all artificial flavorings, colorings, and artificial sweeteners at all costs. Instead, seek out whole foods, locally-grown foods that are in season.

☐ Start reducing all sugars intake and some refined grains with a goal of eliminating them altogether later. For severe scoliosis over 40 degrees or progressive curves over 20 degrees during teenage growing stage I recommend eliminating all grains.

☐ Determine your Metabolic Type® using the questionnaire outlined in the book, **The Metabolic Typing Diet: Customize Your Diet to Your Own Unique Body Chemistry** and eat accordingly. This will tell you which foods and in what proportions you should eat for your unique biochemistry. I recommend finding a nutritional advisor familiar with Metabolic Typing® will be able to do a more accurate computerised test.

☐   Make sure you consume enough healthy fats, including those from animal sources, increasing your intake of omega-3 fats and reducing your intake of omega-6 fats from vegetable and seed oils.

☐   Learn to make some form of traditionally fermented foods and start consuming these on a regular basis. This will help to restore your digestive health and the ability to absorb the foods that you eat.

☐   Begin to enjoy fermented foods like kefir and cultured veggies. Kefir and sauerkraut are the easiest to make, while kimchi and natto require a bit more time and effort.

☐   Make it a point to stand out in the sun for 10 to 15 minutes every day. The objective is to develop a healthy tan without getting burned!

Beginners Exercise Plan

☐   Map out the muscle tightnesses based on your scoliosis on page 198 (Fig. 13). Then map out your symptoms using the key provided on page 200 (Fig. 15).

☐   Find trigger points throughout the muscle groups of your body and start working on them based on the procedures on page 287. Use body diagram on page 289 (Fig. 59) to record the trigger points you find.

☐   Once you have mapped out your scoliosis on page 198 (Fig. 13), you will have developed a good idea of which of your spinal muscles feel tight. Begin by going through each stretching and strengthening exercise in the book customized to your scoliosis.

☐   If you are unsure of which exercises to do, then it is advised to try each exercise as described on both sides of the body to find out what areas are tight, need to be stretched more, or which muscles are weak and need to be strengthened.

☐ Start a regular exercise routine of at least 30 minutes every day, starting with stretching and then moving on to your core stability tests and body balancing exercises.

☐ Start by stretching the tight and strengthening the weak muscles from Chapters 14, 15 and 16, while monitoring for improvement with each exercise session. An exercise journal may be useful in this situation. Over time, try to achieve the same level of flexibility and strength on both the sides of the body.

☐ Initially, if the exercises are too overwhelming, then try swimming on a regular basis. It is one of the best exercises for scoliosis and a great way to get your daily dose of vitamin D from the sun.

Advanced Nutritional Plan

☐ Familiarize yourself with foods that are appropriate for your Metabolic Type®. Photocopy the shopping list on page 320 and cross off any foods you may dislike or to which you're allergic. Make 4 copies of the list. Post one on the refrigerator, keep one in the office, and one in your car. For shopping, carry one in your wallet or purse. Look through the shopping list often and soon you will know it off by heart.

☐ Fill out the diet record sheet on page 328 about two to three hours after your meal. Basically, your body communicates to you in three different ways: 1) Through your appetite and cravings, 2) Through your energy levels, and 3) Through your mental and emotional well-being. Within a couple of hours after eating the correct foods for your Metabolic Type®, you should feel better than the way you felt before you ate them.

☐ Fine tune your diet. If you consistently experience negative reactions to a given meal, gradually increasing the amount of protein and fat in that meal each day. If you find that there is a worsening of symptoms or no improvement, reduce your protein and fat intake to where you started from, and instead try increasing the amount of carbohydrates you consume.

☐   By now your skin should be more used to being in the sun on a regular basis. Now increase the time spent tanning to 30 minutes. Morning or afternoon sun is the best for this purpose to avoid intense midday rays.

Advanced Exercise Plan

☐   Core stability is very important for your spine. We have already divided that section into a beginner's and advanced level exercise program. Begin by assessing your core stability at the beginner level first. If your core stability is very weak, continue to practice the assessment until it is done with ease before moving on to the advanced core stability exercises. Remember, the goal is not to obtain a six-pack, as the abdominals are merely one of the many muscle groups which constitute the core. For the core to be strong, all of your muscles must be balanced to provide proper support to your spine.

☐   Ideally, you should practice all the body alignment exercises in front of a mirror or in the presence of another person, who can watch over you and record the progress that you are making.

☐   Increase the difficulty level of the exercises by adding more weight or an unstable surface, like a balance or wobble board.

☐   When you hit an exercise plateau, don't panic. It doesn't necessarily mean you need to work harder or spend more time exercising. Try mixing it up by varying your workout routine. Try new cardiovascular activities, or use free weights if you always use machines for strength training. Changes in your routine will surprise the body and force it to adapt, bringing you to new levels of fitness.

☐ It is important to use exercise equipment detailed in Chapter 17 for the best possible result. For mild curves less than 20 degrees I recommend an Inversion Table. For curves greater than 20 degrees I recommend a Dynamic Brace System and a Vibration Machine which can be purchased through a health care practitioner or contacting the manufacturer found in the readers resource.

☐ Give yourself at least 6 months of exercising and eating your metabolically correct diet before assessing your progress either by taking photos before and after or an X-ray if recommended by your doctor. More than likely correction will be slow, but with persistence and self determination you will get there.

CHAPTER 19

Readers Resource

The following books, websites, organizations and equipment that may be of interest to people with scoliosis. You are also invited to peer into the last part of this book, which lists all the reference sources I used to write this book. There you will find the titles of many more articles and books that pertain to spinal health.

Spinal Correction Centre

Dr. Kevin Lau

302 Orchard Road #06-03
Singapore 238862
Telephone: (+65) 6884 9820

Email: **drkevinlau@gmail.com**
Website: **www.HIYH.info**
Blog: http://drkevinlau.blogspot.com

Call or email enquiry into our in clinic scoliosis correction program or professional Metabolic Typing® assessment with Dr. Kevin Lau.

Information for People Who Don't Live in Singapore

Patients travel from all over South East Asia to the Spinal Correction Centre in Singapore. For the scoliosis correction program the initial patient visit must be on-site, in order to do a comprehensive physical exam, which is required for all new patients. There are six additional appointments that are hands-on sessions and need to be performed in the office as well. After these six visits have been completed in our office, you may have all future sessions with Dr. Kevin Lau by phone while doing the scoliosis correction at home with the neccessary equipment. There are some cases, however, where it may be recommended that a patient return to the office.

Metabolic Typing® assessment can be done over email or phone. In this first of multiple sessions, you will review the results of your Metabolic Typing® questionnaire with Dr. Lau. During this process of discovery, you will receive feedback on how food can make a direct impact on your health and how to create simple changes that will form the foundation on which to build your new healthy lifestyle for years to come. Also nutritional factors that may lead to your scoliosis will be discussed.

If you would like to find out more about other Health In Your Hands products such as the exercise DVD, audiobook and ScolioTrack for iPhone go to **www.HIYH.info.**

Books

The Metabolic Typing Diet: Customize Your Diet to Your Own Unique Body Chemistry

William L. Wolcott, with Trish Fahey

In The Metabolic Typing Diet, Wolcott and acclaimed science writer Trish Fahey provide simple self-tests that you can use to discover your own Metabolic Type® and determine what kind of diet will work best for you. It might be a low-fat, high carbohydrate diet filled with pasta and grains, or a high-fat, high-protein diet focused on meat and seafood, or anything in between. By detailing exactly which foods and food combinations are right for you, *The Metabolic Typing Diet* at last reveals the secret to shedding unwanted pounds and achieving optimum vitality with lasting results.

Dr. Mercola's Total Health Program: The Proven Plan to Prevent Disease and Premature Aging, Optimize Weight and Live Longer

Dr. Joseph Mercola

Featuring world-renowned natural health physician Dr. Joseph Mercola's dietary program in Part One and over 150 healthy and delicious new recipes in Part Two. Designed to help prevent disease, premature aging, optimize weight, increase energy, and love what you eat while doing so. Mercola's easy to follow program will help you avoid and eliminate the underlying causes of health and weight issues.

Nutrition and Physical Degeneration

Dr. Weston A. Price

For nearly 10 years, Weston Price and his wife traveled around the world in search of the secret to health. Instead of looking at people afflicted with disease symptoms, this highly-respected dentist and dental researcher chose to focus on healthy individuals, and challenged himself to understand how they achieved such amazing health. Dr. Price traveled to hundreds of cities in a total of 14 different countries in his search to find healthy people. He investigated some of the most remote areas in the world. He observed perfect dental arches, minimal tooth decay, high immunity to tuberculosis and overall excellent health in those groups of people who ate their indigenous foods. He found when these people were introduced to modernized foods, such as white flour, white sugar, refined vegetable oils and canned goods, signs of degeneration quickly became quite evident.

The Body Ecology Diet

Donna Gates

The Body Ecology Diet is geared to one fundamental law of nature: the fact that our digestive systems are intimately linked to our immune, endocrine, circulatory and central nervous systems. Profoundly affecting all these interlocking systems is an amazing world of benevolent bacteria: the microscopic "good guys" that must be present in your intestines for you to be healthy. Learn more about the importance of kefir, sauerkraut and other fermented foods that help restore and maintain the important "inner ecology" your body needs to function properly and to eliminate or control the symptoms that rob you of the joy of living.

The UV Advantage

Michael Holick, M.D., Phd.

This is the provocative, groundbreaking and potentially bestselling book about the powerful health benefits from the sun. Just as Dr. Atkins was ahead of the curve for years regarding his now-famous diet while mainstream doctors remained skeptical, Dr. Holick has been the leading exponent of formulated sun exposure, going against the grain of the medical establishment. While too much sun can cause wrinkles and raises other health concerns, a LACK of proper sun exposure, our primary source of Vitamin D can cause serious health problems, such as osteoporosis, certain cancers, high blood pressure, Type 1 diabetes, multiple sclerosis, and depression.

The Cholesterol Myth: Exposing the Fallacy that Saturated Fat and Cholesterol Cause Heart Disease

Dr. Uffe Ravnskov

Dr. Ravnskov is the author of numerous articles published in major medical journals. This book elaborates on the lack of connection between diet, blood cholesterol levels and heart disease and questions the widespread use of cholesterol-lowering drugs. Anyone who has been told to go on a low fat diet or take cholesterol-lowering drugs should read this book first and then give it to his or her doctor!

Organization

The Weston A. Price Foundation

PMB Box 106-380
4200 Wisconsin Avenue, NW
Washington, DC 20016

Email: info@westonaprice.org
Website: www.westonaprice.org

The Weston A. Price Foundation is a non-profit nutrition education organization dedicated to continuing Dr. Price's work and returning nutrient-dense foods to our diet. Their website is filled with scientifically sound articles on the benefits of traditional foods based on research untainted by agribusiness and pharmaceutical industry money.

Price-Pottenger Nutrition Foundation

7890 Broadway
Lemon Grove, CA 91945
U.S.A.

Email: info@ppnf.org
Website: www.ppnf.org

PPNF is dedicated to the principle that diets of healthy primitive and non-industrialized peoples must be our guide to healthy living in the 21st Century. The Foundation's most important obligation is to preserve and disseminate the research of Price and Pottenger, to protect it against misuse or misinterpretations, and to collect, coordinate, and disseminate historical, anthropological and scientific information on nutrition, diet, and health, from preconception care through geriatrics.

Websites

www.HIYH.info or www.Scoliosis.com.sg

For more information on the personalised scoliosis correction program with Dr Kevin Lau and about the companion Exercise DVD, Audiobook and ScolioTrack App for iPhone.

www.Mercola.com

Dr. Mercola's website contains over 50,000 pages of useful articles and information on virtually any health topic you are interested in. It is one of the world's most visited natural health website and a site that I regularly go to for reliable health information.

www.NaturalNews.com

The NaturalNews Network is a non-profit collection of public education websites covering topics that empower individuals to make positive changes in their health, environmental sensitivity, consumer choices and informed skepticism.

www.MetabolicTyping.com

This is a key web portal on customized nutrition for health consumers as well as health professionals. Here you'll find a wealth of information related to Metabolic Typing®, including news, features, success stories, and important tips to help you manage your diet and achieve a whole new level of health and fitness.

www.HealthExcel.com

As a research-based organization since 1987, Healthexcel is the established leader in the rapidly emerging field of Metabolic Typing™, or customized nutrition. The company offers advanced computer-based services that enable health professionals to evaluate the highly individualized dietary needs of patients and clients, and to provide customized dietary programs for one's metabolic type.

Equipment

Meditrac Medical Equipment Ltd. (Dynamic Brace System)

53 Pinkas st.
Tel-Aviv 62261
Israel
E-mail: info@meditrac.co.il
Website: www.meditrac.co.il

Meditrac's team of medical researchers and advisors is in the forefront of spine treatment technology. The results of their efforts have led to the development of effective, innovative products, benefiting health care professionals and their patients around the world. I personally use the Vertetrac and Dynamic Brace System on my scoliosis patients in clinic and have personally seen the effectiveness in treating a wide range of spinal conditions. *Email them and mention this book for a special offer.*

Shopping List		
	Carbohydrate Type	**Protein Type**
Meats/Fowl	**Light Meats:** Chicken Breast, Turkey Breast, Lean Pork, Ham, occasional red meat or restrict entirely.	**High Purine:** Organ Meats, Pate, Beef Liver, Chicken Liver, Pork Liver **Medium Purine:** Beef, Bacon, Chicken Thigh, Duck, Fowl, Goose, Kidney, Lamb, Pork Chop, Spare Rib, Turkey, Veal, Wild Game.
Seafood	**Light Fish:** Catfish, Cod, Flounder, Haddock, Halibut, Perch, Scrod, Sole, Trout, Tuna, Turbot	**High Purine:** Anchovy, Caviar, Herring, Mussel, Sardine **Medium Purine:** Abalone, Clam, Crab, Crayfish, Lobster, Mackerel, Octopus, Oyster, Salmon, Scallop, Shrimp, Squid
Eggs	Chicken Eggs, Quail Eggs	Chicken Eggs, Quail Eggs, Fish Roe, Caviar.
Dairy	**Non/Low Fat:** Cheese, Cottage Cheese, Cow Or Goats Milk, Kefir, Homemade Yogurt	**Full Fat:** Cow Or Goats Milk, *Kefir*, Homemade Yogurt, Soft Cheese, Cream, Cottage Cheese
Fats	Use Sparingly **For cooking:** Ghee (clarified butter), Extra virgin coconut oil, Coconut milk (canned), Butter from goats or cow **For salads (not for cooking):** Extra Virgin Olive Oil, Flaxseed Oil, Hempseed Oils, Nut Oils, Seed Oils	All Okay **For cooking:** Ghee (clarified butter), Extra virgin coconut oil, Coconut milk (canned), Butter from goats or cow **For salads (not for cooking):** Extra Virgin Olive Oil, Flaxseed Oil, Hempseed Oils, Nut Oils, Seed Oils

Table 3: Shopping list for each Metabolic Type®.

	Carbohydrate Type	Protein Type
Vegetables	**High Glycemic Index:** Potatoes, Pumpkin, Rutabaga, Sweet Potato, Yam **Moderate Glycemic Index:** Beet, Corn, Eggplant, Okra, Parsnip, Radish, Squash, Zucchini **Low Glycemic Index:** Beet Green, Broccoli, Brussel Sprouts, Cabbage, Chard, Collard, Cucumber, Garlic, Kale, Kai-Lang And Other Asian Greens, Leafy Greens, Onion, Parsley, Peppers, Scallion, Sprouts, Tomato, Watercress.	**Non-Starch:** Asparagus, Beans (fresh), Cauliflower, Celery, Mushroom, Spinach. **Moderate Glycemic Index:** Artichoke, Carrot, Pea, Potatoes (Fried In Butter Only), Squash.
Fruits	**High Glycemic Index:** Banana, Mango, Papaya, Durian, Lychee and other Tropical Fruits. **Moderate Glycemic Index:** Apples, Apricots, Grapes, Melon, Peaches, Pears, Oranges, Plums, Pineapple, Kiwi, Dragon Fruit, Passion Fruit, Pomegranates, Guava. **Low Glycemic Index:** Blueberries, Blackberries, Strawberrys, Raspberries, Grapefruit, Lemon, Lime, Cherry, Green Apple, Young Green Coconuts (meat only).	**High Glycemic Index:** Not Fully Ripe Banana **Low Glycemic Index:** Avocado, Olives, Not Fully Ripe Apples or Pears.

Table 3: Shopping list for each Metabolic Type®.

10 Easy Ways to Shop for Healthy Foods at Your Local Supermarket

We've all done it before. We're late. We've had a long day at work and there's no food in the house, so we quickly dash through the supermarket like we're contestants on Supermarket Sweep and throw whatever we need in the shopping cart and get out.

Well, it's in these reckless binge runs that we can do our bodies harm by carelessly throwing whatever comes to hand first into our carts. We usually grab food items that easy to make and that tastes good. Unfortunately these items tend to be highly processed foods packed with sugar and sodium!

Now, if you're like most people, you probably think you don't have the time or money to spend buying healthy foods, or you think if you want to eat healthy you need to go to a special health food store to shop. Well, throw all those excuses out the window. Your local grocery store packs on average about 40,000 items and many of these are healthy alternatives to what's in your shopping cart.

So get ready as we show you 10 ways to easily shop for healthy foods without breaking your budget or wasting time looking for a health food store.

1. **Shop with a List!**

   Don't just wander aimlessly through the store. Know what you need and keep it neatly organized on a list you can easily read while shopping. Spending just a little time each day putting together this list will save you time later when you are actually in the grocery store. It also helps if you know your grocery store and categorize your items by the department they can be found in. This way you can avoid backtracking through the store when you realize your forgot something back in the dairy aisle. Keeping a list also prevents you from succumbing to the junk food aisle, saving you from unhealthy foods that are full of empty calories and sugar.

2. **Don't Shop on an Empty Stomach!**

    You know this is a bad idea. Once you hit the aisles and your stomach starts growling, you're liable to pick up anything you see! By making sure you shop for food on a full stomach, you'll eliminate buying foods that are bad for you as well as food you just don't need. This saves your body and your wallet. If you can't shop after a meal, make sure you at least drink a glass of water before you go in to help alleviate some of your hunger.

3. **Buy Fresh Food!**

    It really can't get any simpler than this when it comes to eating healthy. By adding fresh foods such as fruits and vegetables to your list, you can easily add the needed vitamins and minerals you need to maintain a healthy diet. Take a look at what you're currently buying. If more than 50 percent of your groceries are coming from a box or a can, you need to reevaluate your choices and head toward the fresh food.

4. **Shop the Perimeter of the Store.**

    When you're searching for the freshest foods, it helps to stay out of the central aisles unless absolutely necessary. In your local grocery store, the perimeter of the store is where they keep all the fresh food items including produce, dairy, and seafood.

5. **Don't Walk By the Organics.**

    When it comes to fresh food, quality counts, and your organics section should be one of your first stops in the grocery store. It may be a little more expensive than the regular section, but the added benefit of not having chemicals and pesticides is well worth the price. If you shop these sections right, you can target the items that are on sale and even get your organic food for less than your non-organics.

6. **Stay Away from Foods and Drinks with Corn Syrup.**

   There is no nutritional value to corn syrup. It's just an empty sweetener that is almost as bad as refined sugar. Don't be fooled! Make sure you read the labels carefully and if corn syrup is one of the first four ingredients, put it down and walk away. You'll be surprised at how many foods are packed with corn syrup including fruit juices, spaghetti sauces, and even some bread.

7. **Fresh Is the Best but Frozen Is Good Too.**

   It's not always feasible to have fresh foods all the time. So when fresh foods aren't available, head toward the frozen aisle for a backup. Frozen vegetables and fruits are most often flash-frozen, which locks in nutrients. It's always a good idea to keep a couple bags of frozen fruits or vegetables in your freezer. You can toss them in the microwave for a quick side dish, make fruit smoothies, or toss into plain yogurt for a fresh fruit taste.

8. **Keep Canned Tomato Products in Your Pantry.**

   Fresh tomatoes are great but here's one exception where fresher actually isn't better. Studies have shown that tomato sauces, crushed tomatoes, and stewed tomatoes actually have an increased amount of the antioxidant lycopene. That's because they are concentrated. Keeping these kitchen jewels handy can help you out the next time you are wondering what's for dinner. Just throw some chicken and sauce in a crock pot or add crushed tomatoes to a soup, and you've got a healthy meal in no time!

9. **Avoid Processed Foods.**

   Remember all those boxes and bags you were throwing in your cart earlier? Most likely it was all processed foods like chips, cookies, and frozen pizza. Save your money and your body. Skip the junk food and stock up on your fruits, vegetables, and meats instead. You'll avoid the sugar rush and feel better in the long run.

10. Try Whole Grains.

The availability of whole grains has increased and it's not uncommon to find whole grain products next to their processed counterpart. Whole grain pastas, brown rice, and whole wheat flour are great alternatives that not only are healthy, but they taste great, too. One warning when it comes to whole wheat products. Because more and more people are reaching for whole grains these days, packaging has gotten a little tricky. For instance, wheat bread is a good alternative to white bread, but look closely next time you pick up a loaf of wheat bread. If the first ingredient is refined wheat flour, then put it back. It's made from the same stuff as white bread and quite possible is dyed brown to make it look healthier. As a general rule, whole wheat breads tend to be heavier and denser than white bread.

You don't have to be a health nut to shop for healthy foods. With just a little discipline and by practicing the steps above, you'll see how easy it is to shop for healthy foods in the comfort of your own local grocery store.

Ingredients to Avoid

It is important to start reading labels on foods. Here is a list of ingredient based on scientific evidence that has been linked to the following disease or disorder. By cutting out all forms of processed foods and moving to a diet that is natural and composed of whole foods, basically all of these dietary dangers can be avoided.

From personal experience, sugar and refined grains seem to be the most difficult food item to eliminate. Gradually, start reducing the intake of, or completely eliminate as in the case for protein types, all grains, beans and legumes. Children with active scoliosis during the growth spurt period or have high fasting insulin (check with a fasting insulin test by doctors) need to diligently eliminate sugar, refined grains and starchy carbohydrates.

Try walking down a supermarket isle and find a product that does not contain at least one of these ingredients. While not impossible, it certainly would be difficult as most food companies regularly add them to improve shelf life or tastes of their products. The easiest solution is to try to eliminate all process foods and start making foods like your great, great grandmother used to with fresh ingredients and whole foods.

Giving up the foods your taste buds love to experience is not always easy. In fact, it is one of the hardest changes to make. Western medicine counts on the fact that most people are inherently lazy. Most people will rather lose their health rather than experience the discomfort and inconvenience required to give up the foods and ingredients that are literally killing them.

Remember: Your body wants to heal itself. All you have to do is give it the foods and physical exercise it needs, and stop poisoning yourself with dangerous food ingredients.

Ingredient	Associated Diseases
Sugar	Obesity, heart disease, mental disorders, hormonal disorders, cancers, diabetes
Refined Grains White Rice, White Flour, Instant Oats	Obesity, heart disease, mental disorders, hormonal disorders, cancers, diabetes
Highly Processed Foods Breads, Pasta, Cereal, Biscuits, French fries, Candy, Ice cream, Chips, Pretzels, Waffles, Pancakes, Baked goods, Donuts	Obesity, heart disease, mental disorders, hormonal disorders, cancers, diabetes
MSG Canned soups, pre-prepared stocks often known as stock cubes, condiments such as barbecue sauce, frozen dinners, common snack foods such as flavored potato chips and biscuits, most fast food.	Parkinson's disease, Alzheimer's disease, heart disorders, reproductive disorders, obesity, growth hormone imbalance, hyperactivity, violent behaviour, asthma, seizures, headaches
Hydrogenated Oils (Margarine, fast foods, processed foods, commercial baked goods, peanut butter).	Cardiovascular heart disease, cancer, diabetes
Sodium Nitrates (Processed meats such as bacon and sausages)	Cancers, especially of the digestive tract
Aspartame (Diet sodas, sugar free gums)	Dizziness, loss of memory, sleep disorders, Blindness, mental confusion, cancer.
Highly Acidic Ingredients Vinegars, soda	Osteoporosis, loss of bone mass, digestive problems

Table 4: Metabolic Disruptors

Diet Record Sheet Date:_____		
Reactions after a meal	**Good**	**Bad**
APPETITE FULLNESS / SATISFACTION SWEET CRAVINGS	Following the meal . . . ☐ Feel full, satisfied ☐ Do NOT have sweet cravings ☐ Do NOT desire more food ☐ Do NOT get hungry soon after ☐ Do NOT need to snack before next meal	Following the meal . . . ☐ Feel physically full, but still hungry ☐ Don't feel satisfied; feel like something was missing from meal ☐ Have desire for sweets ☐ Feel hungry again soon after meal ☐ Need to snack between meals
ENERGY LEVELS	Normal energy response to meal: ☐ Energy is restored after eating ☐ Have good, lasting, "normal" sense of energy and well-being	Poor energy response to meal: ☐ Too much or too little energy ☐ Become hyper, jittery, shaky, nervous, or speedy ☐ Feel hyper, but exhausted "underneath" ☐ Energy drop, fatigue, exhaustion, sleepiness, drowsiness, lethargy, or listlessness
MENTAL EMOTIONAL WELL-BEING	Normal qualities: ☐ Improved well-being ☐ Sense of feeling refueled and restored ☐ Upliftment in emotions ☐ Improved clarity and acuity of mind ☐ Normalization of thought processes	Abnormal qualities: ☐ Mentally slow, sluggish, spacey ☐ Inability to think quickly or clearly ☐ Hyper, overly rapid thoughts ☐ Inability to focus/hold attention ☐ Hypo traits: Apathy, depression, sadness ☐ Hyper traits: Anxious, obsessive, fearful, angry, short tempered, or irritable, etc.

Table 5: Diet Record Sheet
(Photocopy and keep in a food diary)

Body Balancing Stretches

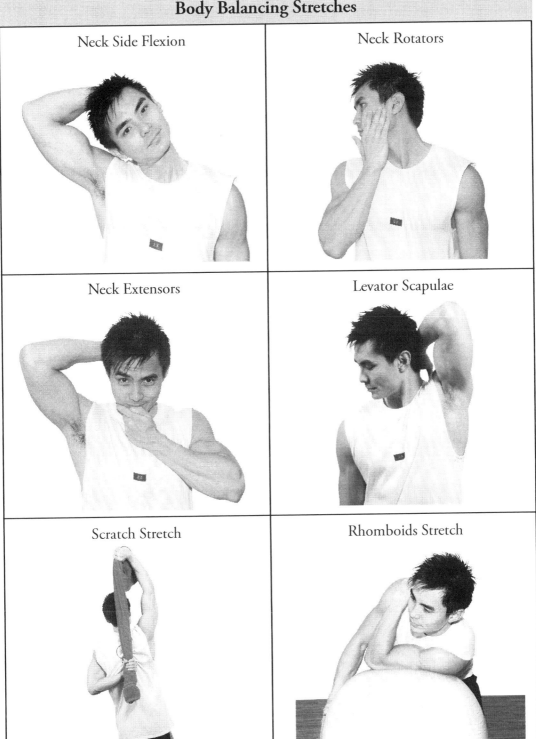

Neck Side Flexion

Neck Rotators

Neck Extensors

Levator Scapulae

Scratch Stretch

Rhomboids Stretch

Body Balancing Stretches (continued)

Overhead Stretch (hands together)	Overhead Stretch (palms inverted)
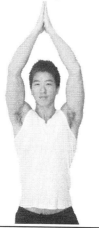	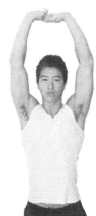
Trunk Side Bending (heel sitting)	Thoracic Side Bending (edge of table)
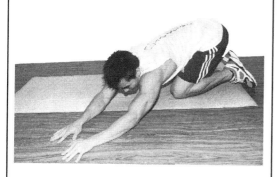	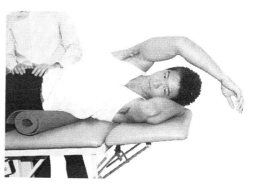
Lumbar Side Bending (edge of table)	Lumbar Scoliosis Stretch
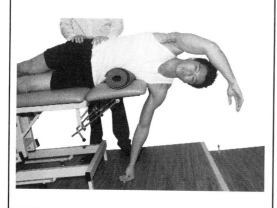	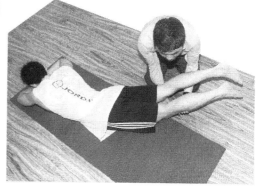

Body Balancing Stretches (continued)

Trunk Rotation

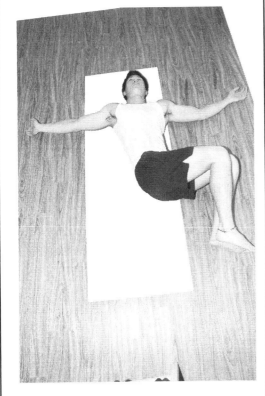

Hamstrings

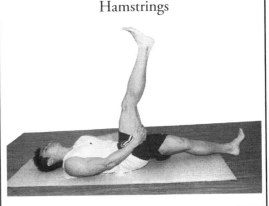

Iliotibial Band

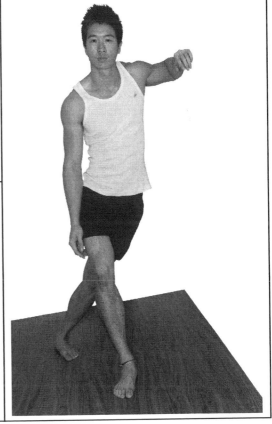

Middle Back and Abdominals

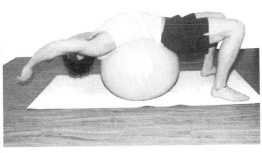

Core Stability Exercises Tests

Level 1: Plank Position

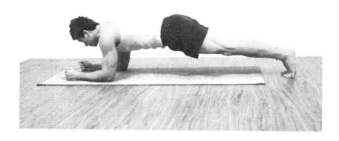

Level 2: Plank Position with Arm Lift

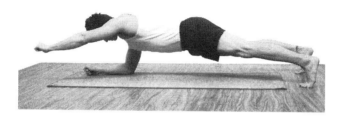

Level 3: Plank Position with Leg Lift

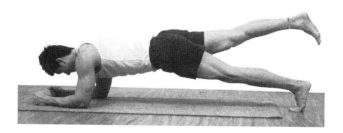

Level 4: Plank with Opposite Leg and Arm Lift

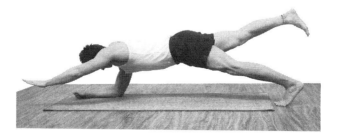

Beginner Core Stability Exercises

Lower Abdominal Conditioning

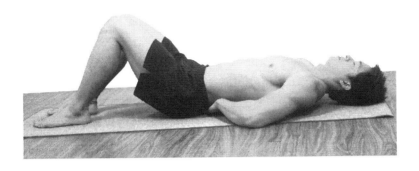

Lower Abdominal Conditioning with Leg Lift

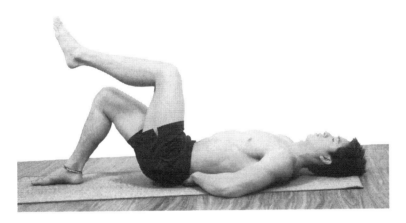

Four-Point Tummy Vacuum

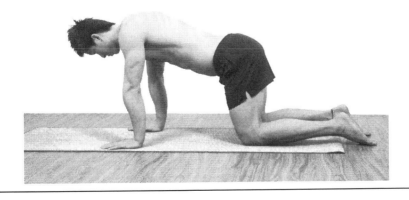

Advanced Core Stability Exercises

Forward Ball Roll

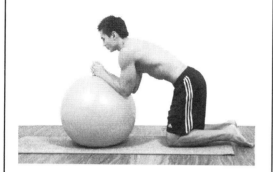

Jack-knife with Ball

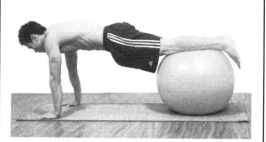

Swiss Ball Crunch

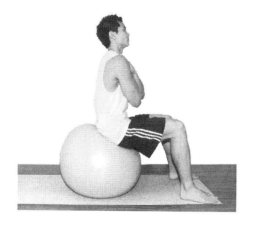

Dynamic Horse Stance

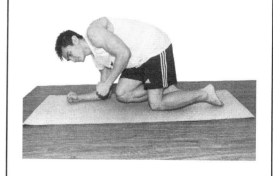

Body Alignment Exercises

Neck Flexion with Ball	Neck Extension with Ball
Neck Side-bend with Ball	Pelvic Rock — Front to Back
Pelvic Rock — Side to Side	Pelvic Rock — Figure 8

Body Alignment Exercises (continued)

Breathing Squats

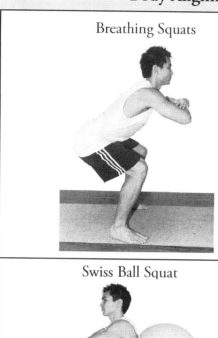

Single Arm Overhead Squat

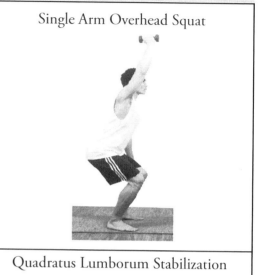

Swiss Ball Squat

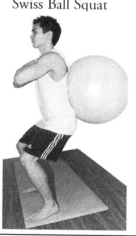

Quadratus Lumborum Stabilization

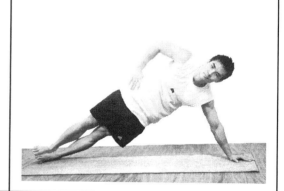

Swiss Ball Side Flexion

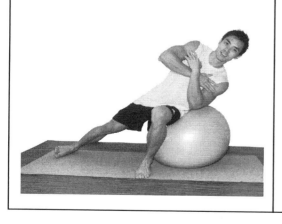

Wall Push Up

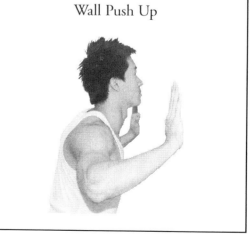

Seated Bend Pull

Final Words

Life is about choices. We make choices every day, some more important than others. Perhaps the most important decisions we make are those concerning our health.

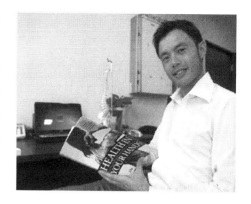

Like many others, you may have wrongly assumed that there is nothing you can do to alter your chances of getting a disease. Nothing can be farther from the truth: your body may have tendencies towards certain diseases or conditions, but it is within your power to change the course of your physical health.

By simply eating properly and adding some form of exercise to your daily routine, you can have a significant impact on whether good or bad genes are expressed. To put it more simply, just because you have a genetic tendency towards heart disease, diabetes or scoliosis does not mean that there is nothing you can do to avoid developing any of these conditions. Eating a nutrient-rich diet and exercising regularly can improve your health and help prevent against the development of disease.

Doctors constantly advise their patients to change their diet and lifestyle. This is because they know that doing so can reduce their patients' chances of succumbing to lifestyle-related conditions, such as obesity, diabetes, heart disease, and even scoliosis.

We have within us the power to modify the expression of our genes. Our genes determine who we are, but not how we are. We can choose to be healthy and decrease our risks of certain diseases to which we may be genetically susceptible.

Eating is one of the basic tenets of our life. I have provided an explanation and a plan for enhancing your genes and health. I encourage you to use this information to make the right choices, the ones that build the foundation for a long and healthy life.

Before I Wind Up….

I hope you have benefited and enjoyed reading this book, as much as I enjoyed putting it together for you. Contained within are information which is as up to date as possible, some research such as the importance of gut health and serotonin in bone formation was discovered during the final editing of this book.

However, our journey on the road to full recovery for your scoliosis is far from over. New techniques and new treatments are being discovered and re-discovered every day.

Should you come across any such treatment, or if you have any recommendation/feedback for improving this book, please do not hesitate to send me your comments at:

scoliosis.feedback@gmail.com

If you would like to find out more about other Health In Your Hands products such as the exercise DVD, audiobook and ScolioTrack for iPhone go to:

www.HIYH.info

I would be most thankful to you for your suggestions and would happily try to incorporate those in the next edition of this book.

Knowledge is power. Use it wisely to promote good health.

Dr Kevin Lau D.C.

References

(Chapter 1 — 7)

**Part 1
Background and
Theory behind
the Program**

1. Brignall, M. (Jun 13, 2002). Diet and Lifestyle Changes Slow Progression of Prostate Cancer, Stopgettingsick.com, http://www.stopgettingsick.com/Conditions/condition_template.cfm/5888/293/1.

2. Null, G. PhD, Dean, C. MD ND, Feldman, M. MD, Rasio, D. MD and Smith, D. PhD. (Oct, 2003). Death By Medicine, Nutrition Institute of America Report, http://www.nutritioninstituteofamerica.net/research/DeathByMedicine/DeathByMedicine1.htm.

3. Jaganathan, J. (Jun 18, 2008). 1 in 10 above age 40 has curved spine disorder, The Straits Times.

4. Nowak, A. and Czerwionka-Szaflarska. M. (1998) Clinical picture of mitral valve proplapse syndrome in children - a study of a self-selected material. Med Sci Monit, 4(2): 280-284

5. Warren M.P., Brooks-Gunn J., Hamilton L.H., Warren L.F.and Hamilton W.G. (1986). Scoliosis and fractures in young ballet dancers: relation to delayed menarche and secondary amenorrhea. N Engl J Med, 314:1348—1353.

6. Akella P., Warren M.P., Jonnavithula S. and Brooks-Gunn J. (Sept, 1991) Scoliosis in ballet dancers. Med Probl Performing Artists. 84—86.

7. Tanchev, P.I., Dzherov, A.D., Parushev, A.D., Dikov, D.M., and Todorov, M.B. (Jun, 2000). Scoliosis in rhythmic gymnasts. Spine, vol 25 (issue 11): 1367-72

8. Omey, M.L., Micheli, L. J. and Gerbino, P.G. (2000). Idiopathic scoliosis and spondylolysis in the female athlete: Tips for treatment. Clinical orthopaedics and related research, 372, 74-84

9. Riseborough E. and Wynne-Davies R. (1973) A genetic survey of idiopathic scoliosis in Boston. J Bone Joint Surg Am, 55:974-982.

10. Czeizel A., Bellyei A., Barta O., et al. (1978) Genetics of adolescent idiopathic scoliosis. J Med Genet, 15:424-427.

11. Farley, D. (Jul, 1994). Correcting the curved spine of scoliosis - includes related article on X-ray safety. FDA Consumer. 28(6):26-29.

12. Bunnell, W.P. (1988) The natural history of idiopathic scoliosis. Clin Orthop. 229:20-25.

13. Weinstein S.L., Zavala D.C. and Ponseti I.V. (Jun, 1981). Idiopathic Scoliosis: long-term follow-up & prognosis in untreated patients. J Bone Joint Surg Am, 63(5): 702-12.

14. Fayssoux, R.S., Cho, R.H. and Herman M.J. (2010) A History of Bracing for Idiopathic Scoliosis in North America Clin Orthop Relat Res, 468:654–64.

15. Coillard C., Circo A.B. and Rivard C.H. (November, 2010) SpineCor treatment for Juvenile Idiopathic Scoliosis: SOSORT award 2010 winner. Scoliosis, 5:25, doi: 10.1186/1748-7161-5-25.

16. Negrini S., Minozzi S., Bettany-Saltikov J., Zaina F., Chockalingam N., Grivas T.B., Kotwicki T., Maruyama T., Romano M. and Vasiliadis E.S. (2010) Braces for idiopathic scoliosis in adolescents. Cochrane Database of Systematic Reviews, Issue 1. Art. No.: CD006850.

17. Dale, E. Rowe, M.D., Saul, M. Bernstein, M.D., Max, F. Riddick, M.D., Adler, F. M.D., Emans. J.B. M.D. and Gardner-Bonneau, D. Ph.D. (May, 1997). A Meta-Analysis of the Efficacy of Non-Operative Treatments for Idiopathic Scoliosis, The Journal of Bone and Joint Surgery 79:664-74.

18. Miller, J.A., Nachemson, A.L. and Schultz, A.B. (Sept, 1984). Effectiveness of braces in mild idiopathic scoliosis. Spine, 9(6):632-5.

19. Nachemson, A.L. and Peterson, L.E. (1995). Effectiveness of treatment with a brace in girls who have adolescent idiopathic scoliosis. A prospective, controlled study based on data from the Brace Study of the Scoliosis Research Society. The Journal of Bone and Joint Surgery, 77(6), 815-822.

20. Dolan L.A. and Weinstein SL. (Phila Pa 1976; Sep, 2007) Surgical rates after observation and bracing for adolescent idiopathic scoliosis: an evidence-based review. Spine, 1: 32(19 Suppl): S91-S100.

21. Ogilvie J., Nelson L., Chettier R. and Ward K. (2009) Does bracing alter the natural history of Adolescent Idiopathic Scoliosis? Scoliosis, 4(Suppl 2): O59.

22. Karol L.A. (Phila Pa 1976; Sep, 2001). Effectiveness of bracing in male patients with idiopathic scoliosis, 26(18): 2001-5.

23. Weiss H.R. (Jan 1, 2001). Adolescent Idiopathic Scoliosis: The Effect of Brace Treatment on the Incidence of Surgery. Spine, 26(1), 42-47.

24. Morningstar M.W., Woggon D. and Lawrence G. (Sep, 2004) Scoliosis treatment using a combination of manipulative and rehabilitative therapy: a retrospective case series. BMC Muculoskelet Disord, 14(5): 32.

25. Dickson, R. A. and Weinstein, S. L. (Mar, 1999). Bracing (And Screening) — Yes Or No?, British Editorial Society of Bone and Joint Surgery, 81(2): 193-8.

26. Farley, D. (Jul, 1994). Correcting the curved spine of scoliosis - includes related article on X-ray safety. FDA Consumer. 28(6):26-29.

27. Humke T., Grob D., Scheier H. and Siegrist H. (1995) Cotrel-Dubousset and Harrington Instrumentation in idiopathic scoliosis: a comparison of long-term results. Eur Spine J, 4(5): 280-3.

28. Mohaideen A., Nagarkatti D., Banta J.V. and Foley C.L. (Feb, 2007) Not all rods are Harrington - an overview of spinal instrumentation in scoliosis treatment. Pediatr Radiol, 30(2): 110-8.

29. Steinmetz M.P., Rajpal S. and Trost G. (Sep, 2008) Segmental spinal instrumentation in the management of scoliosis. Neurosurgery, 63(3 Suppl): 131-8.

30. Margulies J.Y., Neuwirth M.G., Puri R., Farcy F.V. and Mirovsky Y. (Apr, 1995) Cotrel Dubousset and Wisconsin segmental spine instrumentation: comparison of results in adolescents with idiopathic scoliosis King Type II. Contemp Orthop, 30(4): 311-4.

31. Sucato D.J. (Phila Pa 1976; Dec, 2010) Management of severe spinal deformity: scoliosis and kyphosis. Spine, 35(25): 2186-92.

32. Shamji M.F. and Isaacs R.E. (Sep, 2008) Anterior-only approaches to scoliosis. Neurosurgery, 63(3 Suppl): 139-48.

33. Wilk B., Karol L.A., Johnston C.E., 2nd, Colby S. and Haideri N. (2006) The Effect of Scoliosis Fusion Surgery on Spinal Ranges of Motion: a Comparison of Fused & Nonfused Patients with Idiopathic Scoliosis. Spine, 31(3): 309-314.

34. Yawn, B.P., Yawn, R.A., Roy A. (Sep 15, 2000). The estimated cost of school scoliosis screening. Spine, 25(18):2387-91.

35. Danielsson, A.J., Wiklund, I. , Pehrsson, K. and Nachemson, A.L. (Aug, 2001). Health-related quality of life in patients with adolescent idiopathic scoliosis: a matched follow-up at least 20 years after treatment with brace or surgery. European Spine Journal. 10(4), 278-288

36. Akazawa1, T., Minami1, S., Takahashi1 K., Kotani1 T., Hanawa T. and Moriya1 H. (Mar, 2005) Corrosion of spinal implants retrieved from patients with scoliosis. J Orthop Sci, 10(2):200-5.

37. Wilk B., MS; Karol L.A., MD; Johnston C.E., II MD; Colby S. and Haideri, N. PhD (Feb 22, 2006). The Effect of Scoliosis Fusion Surgery on Spinal Ranges of Motion: a Comparison of Fused & Nonfused Patients with Idiopathic Scoliosis. Spine, 31(3):309-314.

38. Weinstein S.L., Dolan L.A., Spratt K.F., Peterson K.K., Spoonamore M.J. and Ponseti I.V. (Feb, 2003) Health and function of patients with untreated idiopathic scoliosis: a 50-year natural history study. JAMA, 289(5): 559-67.

39. Götze C., Liljenqvist U.R., Slomka A., Götze H.G. and Steinbeck J. (Jul, 2002) Quality of life and back pain: outcome 16.7 years after Harrington instrumentation. Spine (Phila Pa 1976), 27(13): 1456-63.

40. Sponseller P.D., Cohen M.S., Nachemson A.L., Hall J.E. and Wohl M.E. (Jun, 1987) Results of surgical treatment of adults with idiopathic scoliosis. J Bone Joint Surg Am, 69(5): 667-75.

41. Akazawa T., Minami S., Takahashi K., Kotani T., Hanawa T. and Moriya H. (2005) Corrosion of spinal implants retrieved from patients with scoliosis. J Orthop Sci, 10(2): 200-5.

42. Bunge E.M. and de Koning, H.J. (Feb, 2009) The effectiveness of screening for scoliosis. Pediatrics for Parents. http://findarticles.com/p/articles/mi_m0816/is_2_25/ai_n31506277/

43. Hawes, M. (2006). Impact of spine surgery on signs and symptoms of spinal deformity. Developmental Neurorehabilitation, 1751-8431, 9(4); 318 — 339.

44. Ogilvie J.W. (Jan-Feb, 2011) Update on prognostic genetic testing in adolescent idiopathic scoliosis (AIS). J Pediatr Orthop, 31(1 Suppl): S46-8.

45. University of Utah (2007, December 11). Are Humans Evolving Faster? Findings Suggest We Are Becoming More Different, Not Alike. *ScienceDaily*. Retrieved Jan 2, 2007, from http://www.sciencedaily.com /releases/2007/12/071210212227.htm

46. Price, W. (1939) Nutrition and Physical Degeneration, sixth ed. Los Angeles: Price-Pottenger Foundation.

47. Opsahl, W., Abbott, U., Kenney, C., and Rucker, R. (July 27, 1984). Scoliosis in chickens: responsiveness of severity and incidence to dietary copper. Science, 225: 440-442.

48. Greve, C., Trachtenberg, E., Opsahl, W., Abbott U. and Rocker, R. (18 Aug, 1986). Diet as an External Factor in the Expression of Scoliosis in a Line of Susceptible Chickens. The Journal of Nutrition, 117: 189-193.

49. Johnston, W.L., MacDonald, E. and Hilton, J.W., (Nov, 1989). Relationships between dietary ascorbic acid status and deficiency, weight gain and brain neurotransmitter levels in juvenile rainbow trout. Fish Physiology and Biochemistry, 6(6): 353-365.

50. Lim, C. and Lovell, R.T. (1977), Pathology of the Vitamin C Deficiency Syndrome in Channel Catfish (Ictalurus punctatus). The Journal of Nutrition, 108: 1137-1146.

51. Machlin, L.J., Filipski, R., J. Nelson, Horn, L.R. and Brin, M. (1977), Effects of a Prolonged Vitamin E Deficiency in the Rat. The Journal of Nutrition, 107: 1200-1208.

52. Halver, J.E., Ashley, L.M., and Smith, R.R. (1969), Ascorbic Acid Requirements of Coho Salmon and Rainbow Trout. Transactions of the American Fisheries Society 98:762—771.

53. Choo, P.S., Smith, T.K., Cho, C. Y. and Ferguson H.W. (1991), Dietary Excesses of Leucine Influence Growth and Body Composition of Rainbow Trout, The Journal of Nutrition, 121: 1932-1939.

54. Lee W.T., Cheung C.S., Tse Y.K., Guo X., Qin L., Ho S.C., Lau J. and Cheng J.C. (2005). Generalized low bone mass of girls with adolescent idiopathic scoliosis is related to inadequate calcium intake and weight bearing physical activity in peripubertal period. Osteoporos Int. 16(9):1024-35.

55. Mantle D, Wilkins RM, Preedy V. A novel therapeutic strategy for Ehlers-Danlos syndrome based on nutritional supplements. Med Hypotheses. 2005;64(2):279-83

56. Worthington V. and Shambaugh P. (1993). Nutrition as an environmental factor in the etiology of idiopathic scoliosis. J Manipulative Physiol Ther., 16(3):169-73.

57. Kolata G., Bone Finding May Point to Hope for Osteoporosis, New York Times, Retrieved 11.12.08 from http://www.nytimes.com.

58. Donovan P. (Mar 21, 2008). Grow Your Own Probiotics, Part 1: Kefir, NaturalNews, Naturalnews.com, http://www.naturalnews.com/022822.html.

59. Neogi T., Booth S.L. and Zhang Y.Q. (2006) Low vitamin K status is associated with osteoarthritis in the hand and knee. Arthritis Rheum, 54:1255—61. PMID: 16572460.

Part 2 Nutritional Program for Health and Scoliosis

(Chapter 8 - 10)

60. Brooks, D. (1 Apr, 2008). India, China lead explosion in diabetes epidemic: researcher, AFP.

61. Child & Family Research Institute (Nov. 21, 2007). Too Much Sugar Turns Off Gene That Controls Effects Of Sex Steroids. ScienceDaily, Retrieved January 9, 2007, from http://www.sciencedaily.com / releases/2007/11/071109171610.htm

62. French, P., Stanton, C., Lawless, F., O'Riordan, E.G., Monahan, F.J., Caffrey, P.J. and Moloney, A.P. (Nov, 2000). Fatty acid composition, including conjugated linoleic acid, of intramuscular fat from steers offered grazed grass, grass silage, or concentrate-based diets. Journal of Animal Science, 78(11); 2849-2855.

63. Resnick, Donald and Niwayama, Gen, *Diagnoses of Bone and Joint Disorders* (Philadelphia: WB Saunders, 1988), p. 758.

64. Jaksic, et al. Plasma proline kinetics and concentrations in young men in response to dietary proline deprivation, *American Journal of Clinical Nutrition*, 1990, 52, 307-312.

65. Gotthoffer, NR, *Gelatin in Nutrition and Medicine* (Graylake IL, Grayslake Gelatin Company, 1945), p. 131

66. Medline abstract of Koyama, et al. Ingestion of gelatin has differential effect on bone mineral density and bodyweight in protein undernutrition, *Journal of Nutrition and Science of Vitaminology*, 2000, 47, 1, 84-86.)

67. Oesser, S, et al. Oral administration of (14) C labeled gelatin hydrolysate leads to an accumulation of radioactivity in cartilage of mice (C57/BL), *Journal of Nutrition*, 1999, 10, 1891-1895.

68. Moskowitz, W, Role of collagen hydrolysate in bone and joint disease, *Seminars in Arthritis and Rheumatism*, 2000, 30, 2, 87-99.

69. Lubec, G, et al. Amino acid isomerisation and microwave exposure, *Lancet*, 1989, 2, 8676, 1392-1393.

70. Davis, Adele, *Let's Get Well* (Signet, 1972), p. 142.

71. Gotthoffer, NR, *Gelatin in Nutrition and Medicine* (Graylake IL, Grayslake Gelatin Company, 1945), pp. 65-68

72. Pottenger, FM, Hydrophilic colloid diet, *Health and Healing Wisdom*, Price Pottenger Nutrition Foundation Health Journal, Spring 1997, 21, 1, 17.

73. Ottenberg, R, Painless jaundice, *Journal of the American Medical Association*, 1935, 104, 9, 1681-1687

74. Reuter Information Service, "Can Gelatin Transmit 'Mad Cow' Disease," *Nando Times*, 1997, www.nando.net

75. Anthony W Norman. (Aug, 2008) A vitamin D nutritional cornucopia: new insights concerning the serum 25-hydroxyvitamin D status of the US population. American Journal of Clinical Nutrition, Vol. 88, No. 6, 1455-1456

76. Goswami, R., Gupta, N., Goswami, D., Marwaha, R.K. and Tandon, N. (Aug 2000). Prevalence and significance of low 25-hydroxyvitamin D concentrations in healthy subjects in Delhi. American Journal of Clinical Nutrition, 72(2), 472-475.

77. Holick M.F. (Sept, 2000). Calcium and Vitamin D. Diagnostics and Therapeutics. Clin Lab Med, 20(3):569-90

78. Tokita, H., Tsuchida, A., Miyazawa, K., Ohyashiki, K., Katayanaqi, S,. Sudo, H., Enomoto, M., Takaqi, Y. and Aoki, T. (2006). Vitamin K2-induced antitumor effects via cell-cycle arrest and apoptosis in gastric cancer cell lines. Int J Mol Med, 17(2):2355-43.

79. Neogi, T., Booth, S.L. and Zhang, Y.Q., et al. (2006). Low vitamin K status is associated with osteoarthritis in the hand and knee. Arthritis Rheum, 54:1255-61.

80. Geleijnse, J.M., Vermeer, C., Grobbee, D.E., Schurgers, L.J., Knapen, M.H.J., Van der Meer, I.M., Hofman, A. and Witteman, J.C.M. (2004). Dietary Intake of Menaquinone Is Associated with a Reduced Risk of Coronary Heart Disease: The Rotterdam Study. J Nutr. 134: 3100-3105.

81. National Health and Medical Research Council. (8 Mar, 2006). Joint Statement and Recommendations on Vitamin K Administration to Newborn Infants to Prevent Vitamin K Deficiency Bleeding in Infancy.

82. Purwosuna, Y., Muharram, Racjam I.A., et al. (Apr, 2006) Vitamin [K_2] treatment for postmenopausal osteoporosis in Indonesia. J Obstet Gynaecol Res, 32:230-4.

Part 3 Body Balancing Stretches and Exercises

(Chapter 11 — 19)

83. Negrini, S., Fusco, C., Minozzi, S., Atanasio, S. Zaina, F. and M. Romano, (2008). Exercises reduce the progression rate of adolescent idiopathic scoliosis: Results of a comprehensive systematic review of the literature. Disability & Rehabilitation. 30(10) ; 772 — 785.

84. Smith, R.M. and Dickson, R.A., (Aug, 1987) Experimental structural scoliosis. The Journal of Bone and Surgery. 69(4):576-81.

85. Bogdanov, O.V., Nikolaeva, N.I. and Mikhaelenok, E.L. (1990). Correction of posture disorders and scoliosis in schoolchildren using functional biofeedback. Zh Nevropatol Psikhiatr Im S S Korsakova, 90(8); 47-9.

86. Woynarowska, B., and Bojanowska, J. (1979) Effect of increased motor activity on changes in posture during puberty. Probl Med Wieku Rozwoj. 8:27-35.

87. Wong, M.S., Mak, A.F., Luk, K.D., Evans, J.H. and Brown, B. (Apr, 2001). Effectiveness of audio-biofeedback in postural training for adolescent idiopathic scoliosis patients. Prosthetics and Orthotics International. 25(1):60-70.

88. Yekutiel, M., Robin G.C. and Yarom R. (1981) Proprioceptive function in children with adolescent idiopathic scoliosis. Spine. 6(6):560-6.

89. Klein, A.C. and Sobel D., (1985). Backache Relief. Times Books.

90. Petruska, G.K. DC, DACRB, A Functional Approach to Treatment of Scoliosis. Retrieved December 19, 2007 from www.doctorpetruska.com.

91. Pećina, M., Daković, M. and Bojanić, I. (1992). The natural history of mild idiopathic scoliosis. Acta Med Croatica. 46(2):75-8.

92. Timgren J & Soinila S. (2006). Reversible pelvic asymmetry: an overlooked syndrome manifesting as scoliosis, apparent leg-length difference, and neurologic symptoms. Journal Manipulative Physiological Therapeutics, ;29(7):561-5.

93. Hawes, M.C. (2002). Scoliosis and the Human Spine, West Press.

94. Mooney, V., Gulick, J. and Pozos, R. (Apr, 2000) A preliminary report on the effect of measured strength training in adolescent idiopathic scoliosis. Journal of Spinal Disorders, 13(2):102-7.

95. Weiss, H.R. (1992). Influence of an in-patient exercise program on scoliotic curve. Journal of Orthopaedic Trauma. 18(3):395-406.

96. Weiss, H.R. (Feb, 2003). Conservative treatment of idiopathic scoliosis with physical therapy and orthoses. Orthopade, 32(2):146-56.

97. Morningstar, M.W., Woggon D., and Lawrence, G. (14 Sept, 2004). Scoliosis treatment using a combination of manipulative and rehabilitative therapy: a retrospective case series. BMC Musculoskelet Disord. 5: 32

98. Athanasopoulos, S., Paxinos T., Tsafantakis, E., Zachariou, K. and Chatziconstantinou, S. (31 August, 1998). The effect of aerobic training in girls with idiopathic scoliosis. Scandinavian Journal of Medicine and Science in Sports, 9(1):36-40.

99. Timgren, J. and Soinila, S. (September, 2006). Reversible pelvic asymmetry: an overlooked syndrome manifesting as scoliosis, apparent leg-length difference, and neurologic symptoms. Journal Manipulative Physiological Therapeutics, ;29(7):561-5.

100. Hawes, M.C., (2002). Scoliosis and the Human Spine, West Press.

Index

A

activator x 78
adams forward bend test 37
advanced glycation end 142
aging 23, 128, 148, 172, 184, 299, 315
amino acids 107 111, 116, 137, 138, 142, 161, 165, 181
anemia 24, 30, 86, 126, 163
antibiotics 7, 25, 26, 113, 114, 117, 139, 140
antioxidant 111, 133, 158, 184, 324
arthritis 81, 122, 161, 164, 167, 172, 184, 208, 286, 291
ayurvedic 65

B

bacteria 78, 84, 98, 102, 104-111, 113, 115, 118, 121, 130, 155, 180-183, 316
birth defects 27, 151
bleeding 30, 31, 184
blood in the urine. see hematuria
blood loss. *see* bleeding
blood type diet 72
body alignment 191, 206, 259, 310, 335, 336, 337
body balancing stretches 213, 329, 330, 331
bone broth 82, 161, 164, 165
bone density 26, 170
brace 44-48, 50, 54-57, 201, 203, 215, 256, 293, 296-298, 303, 311

C

calcium 31, 33, 85-87, 100, 116, 121-123, 128, 129, 132, 161, 162, 164, 165, 169-172, 181, 183, 346
cancer 24, 25, 33, 78, 85, 88, 108, 125, 128, 135, 140, 146-149, 152, 164, 166, 168, 170, 174, 177, 183, 316, 327
carbohydrates 17, 61, 6-69, 90, 92, 99, 107, 125-135, 137, 138, 142, 149, 183, 310, 314, 320, 326
carbohydrate types 67, 133, 138
cervical spine 192-193
chiropractor 8, 22, 39, 60, 94, 191, 237, 259, 261, 276, 284, 302, 306
cholesterol 22, 64, 69, 91, 110, 141, 150, 179, 317
cobb angle 34, 41, 42, 45, 47, 201, 261
coconuts 99, 150, 151, 171, 321
cod liver oil 155, 173-175
colitis 164
complications. *see* spinal surgery
copper 99, 100, 101
core 17, 33, 120, 144, 190, 216, 239-253, 255-257, 309, 310, 332-334

Cotrel-Dubousset 49, 50
Crohn's 112, 164
cultured vegetables 107, 110, 118, 119, 182, 183

D

D'Adamo, Peter 72
degenerative diseases 24, 76, 78, 88, 92, 98, 104, 132, 150
depression 5, 8, 84, 104, 146, 152, 316, 328
destructive eating patterns 88
detoxification 22, 24, 162
diabetes 5, 22, 24, 64, 72, 78, 89, 93, 125, 129, 131, 140, 148, 149, 316, 327, 338, 345
disc 24, 44, 88, 132
digestion 74, 92, 98, 102-104, 108, 110, 118, 142, 162, 163, 164, 182
digestive problems 7, 9, 64, 84, 103, 327
down syndrome 29
dynamic brace system 293, 296-298, 311

E

emotional stress 88, 285
ergonomics 191, 207

F

fad diets 61, 137
fermented 17, 82, 89, 98, 105, 107-111, 119, 121, 155, 158, 180, 181, 308, 316

fibromyalgia 287
fitness conditioning 190
flexibility 48, 190, 202, 216, 282, 294, 309

G

gelatin 161-166, 347
genetic 22, 28, 32, 35, 44, 56, 62-76, 78, 93, 102-104, 206, 208
glycemic index 134, 135, 321
glycine 161, 162, 164, 165
Goswami, Ravinder 169

H

hamstrings 237, 235, 294, 331
hardware injury 53
harrington rod 50
HDL 150
healthexcel 319
heart disease 28, 29, 69, 89, 91, 110, 125, 128, 130, 141, 145-149, 152, 177, 317, 327, 338, 347
hematuria 30
herbicide 89
hereditary 35, 56, 68
hippocrates 23, 107
holistic nutrition 9
hormonal imbalances 28
hypermobility 31
hypertension 5, 22
hypoestrogenism 30, 31, 32
hypoglycemia 131

I

idiopathic 27, 29, 33, 45, 47, 100, 201, 207, 260, 261, 341-344
iliotibial band 215, 236, 331
infection 49, 52, 70, 140,

152, 174
infertility 85
inuit 149
inversion table 293, 294, 311

J

joint pain 161, 286, 306

K

kefir 89, 108, 110-117, 133, 155, 180, 308, 316, 347
kidneys 22, 90, 97, 125, 163, 182

L

LDL 83, 150
levator scapulae 194, 224, 329
low estrogen levels.. *see* hypoestrogenism
lower back pain 171, 202, 269, 286
lumbar spine 192, 230,
lung 36, 51, 90, 97, 135, 149, 168, 293, 298

M

magnesium 29-31, 101, 116, 128, 129, 161, 164, 181
manganese 99, 100, 101
massage 2, 21, 64, 106, 286, 288, 298, 303
menopause 31, 72
menstruating 30, 31
metabolic typing 23, 62, 67-76, 93, 135, 306, 313, 319
mitral valve prolapse 29, 31
mixed types 65, 67, 133, 138

muscular dystrophy 27

N

natto 89, 108, 110, 121-124, 155, 184, 308
neck extensors 223, 329
neck rotators 222, 329
nerve damage 52, 201
nutrients 1, 23, 93, 109, 121, 124, 123, 135, 138, 141, 146, 151, 152, 153, 160, 161, 164, 182, 324
nutritional imbalances 99, 100, 102, 206

O

obesity 62, 71, 88, 92, 110, 129, 140, 148, 327, 338
omega-3 89, 142, 146, 178, 179
omega-6 89, 146, 178, 179, 308
orthopedic 21, 45, 55, 101
osteoarthritis... *see* arthritis
osteopenia 29, 30, 31, 100
osteoporosis 29-31, 79, 87, 99, 104, 126, 132, 147, 163, 168-172, 183, 208, 306, 348

P

pectus excavatum 32
pesticides 89, 90, 127, 135, 152, 160, 324
pilates 216
post-menopausal 31
posture 36, 189, 191, 205-211, 221, 225, 279, 281, 294, 304
posture retraining 205
Pottenger, Dr. Francis Marrion 105, 164, 318

pregnancy 72, 153, 172, 178

Price, Weston A. 63, 69, 77-85, 97, 151, 175, 181, 315, 317

probiotics 98, 107, 121, 118, 179, 180, 345

processed foods 8, 77, 78, 83-85, 98, 127, 158, 181, 307, 322, 324-327

proline 158, 161-165

protein types 134, 138, 326

pseudoarthrosis 52

psoas 195

puberty 32, 72, 79, 85, 143, 201, 350

R

red meat 91, 138, 320

rhomboids 195, 226, 329

rickets 31, 32,169

S

sacrum and coccyx 192

salt 74, 82, 92, 109, 120, 129, 171

saturated fats 90, 145-150, 313

scoliosis home screen 38, 40, 307

scoliosis research society 46, 342

self assessments 13

serotonin 103, 116, 339

simple carbohydrates 125, 128, 134

skeletal deformity 33

spinal cord injuries 27, 50

spinal surgery 21, 43, 48, 52

spinecor 45

stretching exercises 214, 218, 220

sugar 7, 8, 64, 79, 84, 85, 88, 89, 92, 97-99, 107, 112, 117, 125-139, 151, 158, 181, 306, 315, 322-327

supplements 8, 9, 76, 102, 152, 157-160, 168, 170-173

T

teenagers 85, 87

thoracic spine 44, 192

toxins 23, 118, 141, 286

traditional vs. modern diets 82

trans fat 99, 127, 134, 147-149

trigger points 285-288

V

vegetarian 8, 86, 111, 138

vibration machine 293-295, 311

vitamin D 31, 63, 85, 151-155, 167-177, 309

vitamin K 30, 31, 78, 101, 122-124, 151-155, 181-185, 347

W

Dr. Roger Williams 69

Bill Wolcott. *see* Wolcott, William

Wolcott, William 9, 62, 65, 76, 314

Y

yoga 216, 257, 290, 294

Z

zinc 32, 87, 97

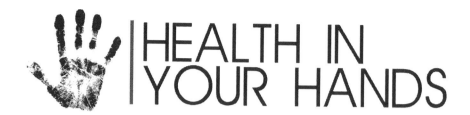

HEALTH IN YOUR HANDS

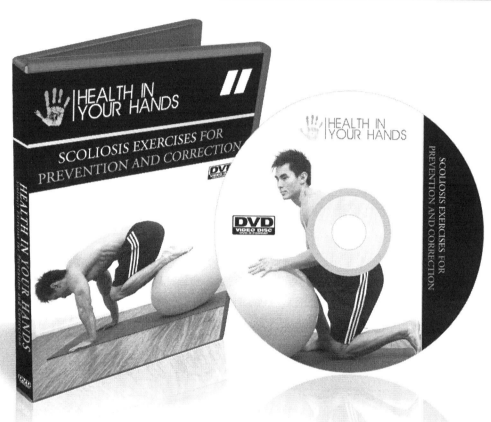

The Health In Your Hands DVD
is a careful selection of exercises that you can do to reverse scoliosis in the comfort of your own home

For anyone who suffers scoliosis, the main advantages of the DVD are:

▶ It gives a 60-minute concise expansion of Dr Lau's book by the same name, Health In Your Hands: Your Plan for Natural Scoliosis Prevention and Treatment.

▶ The Body Balancing section in the DVD explains in detail the correct stretching techniques for scoliosis sufferers to relieve stiffness.

▶ The Building Your Core section focuses on strengthening the muscles that give stability to your spine. Body Alignment Exercises will improve the overall alignment of your spine.

▶ All the exercises that feature in the DVD are suitable for pre and post-operative rehabilitation for scoliosis conditions.

▶ Safe even for those in pain.

▶ All exercises covered in the Health In Your Hands DVD can be practiced at home, and with no special equipment required.

ScolioTrack

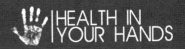

HEALTH IN YOUR HANDS

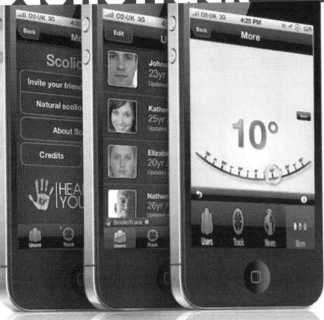

Scoliotrack is a safe and innovative way to track a person's scoliosis condition month to month by using the iPhone accelerometer just as a doctor would with a scoliometer. A scoliometer is an instrument that is used to estimate the amount of curve in a person's spine. It may be used as a tool during screening or as follow-up for scoliosis, a deformity in which the spine curves abnormally.

Features of program

- Can be used with multiple users and saves their data conveniently on the iphone for future checkups

- Tracks and saves a person's Angle of Trunk Rotation (ATR), a key measurement in screening for and planning treatment of scoliosis.

- Tracks a person's height and weight – ideal for growing teenagers with scoliosis or adults who are health conscious.

- Scoliosis progression is graphed making it easy to read month to month changes to a persons scoliosis.

- Displays the latest news feed for scoliosis to keep users informed and up-to-date.

- Full help and easy to follow guides so anyone can track their scoliosis in the comfort of their own home

---

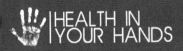
HEALTH IN YOUR HANDS

Audiobook

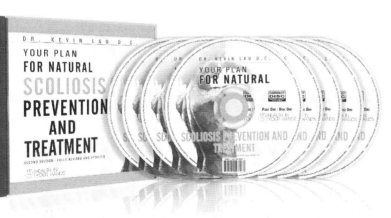

Same information that's in Health In Your Hands – Your Plan for Natural Scoliosis Prevention and Treatment now Unabridged Audiobook package. Narrated by a professional voice talent based in Hollywood USA, the audiobook presents the information in an easy to understand format and convenient format. Spread over 8 CD or approx 8 hours of listening time, Health in Your Hands audiobook allows anyone with a busy schedule to learn the program on the go while driving, exercising or during rest.

For more information for the DVD, ScolioTrack or Audiobook visit: **www.HIYH.info**

Notes

Notes

Follow Us

Stay connected with the latest health tips, news and updates from Dr. Lau with the following social media sites. Join the Health In Your Hands page on Facebook to have the opportunity to ask Dr Kevin Lau questions about the book, general questions about their scoliosis, iPhone App called ScolioTrack or the exercise DVD:

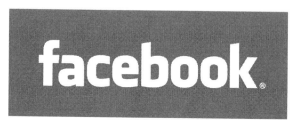

www.facebook.com/HealthInYourHands

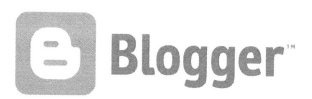

www.DrKevinLau.blogspot.com

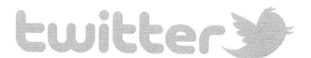

www.twitter.com/DrKevinLau

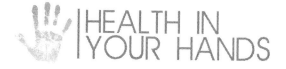

12130117R00192

Made in the USA
Charleston, SC
14 April 2012